Heart Valve Surgery

Edited by Sameh M. Said and Jeffrey Shuhaiber

Published in London, United Kingdom

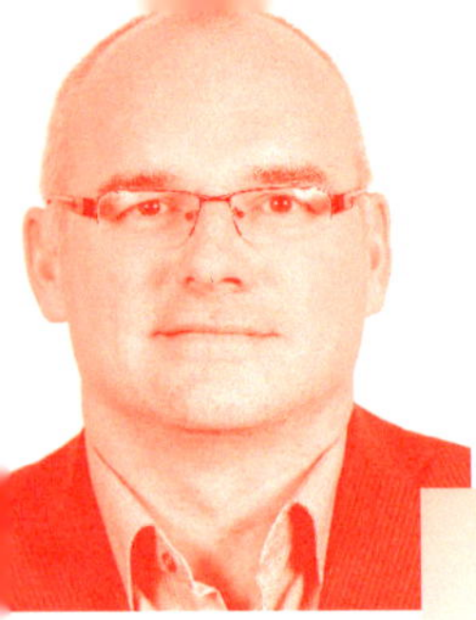
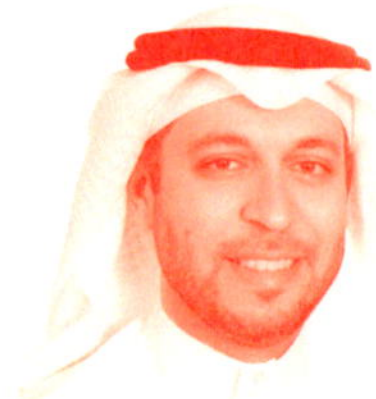
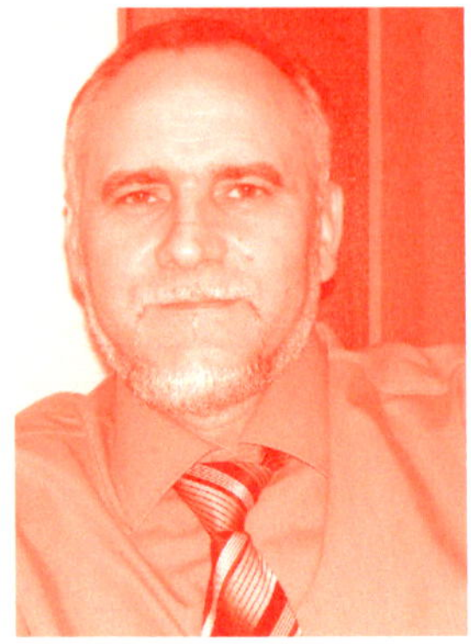
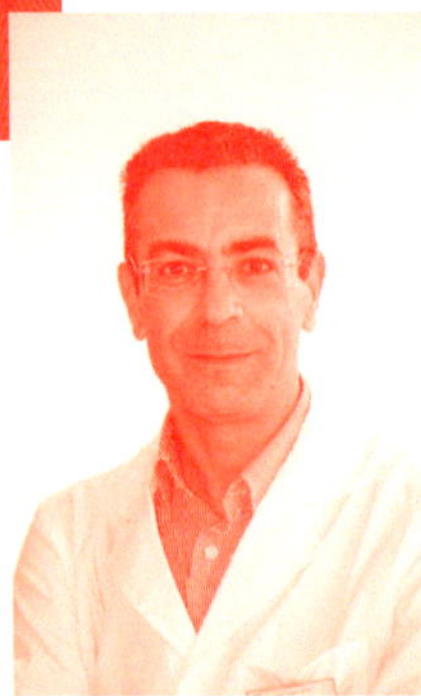
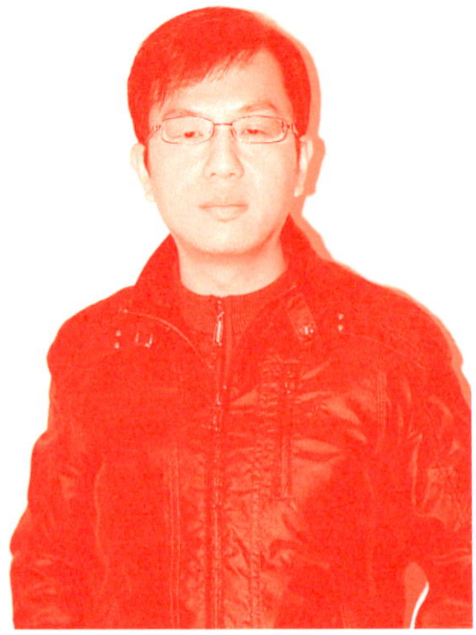
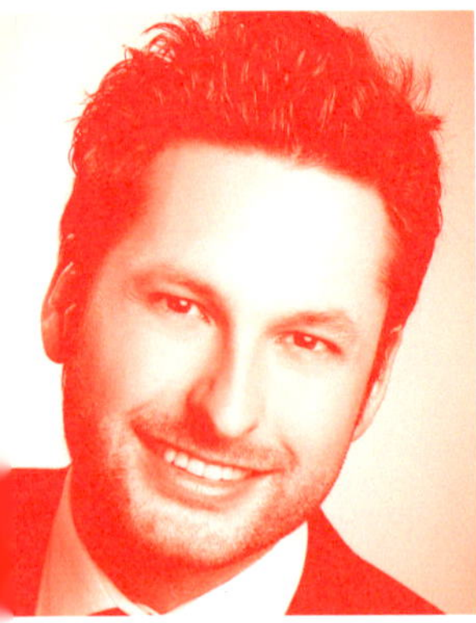
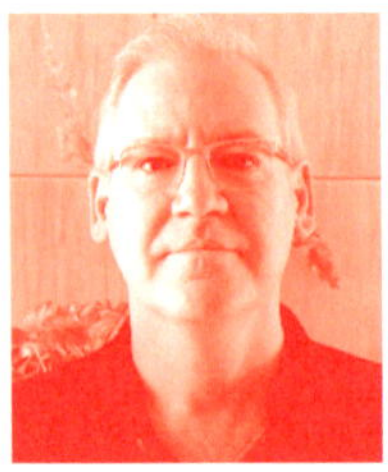

IntechOpen

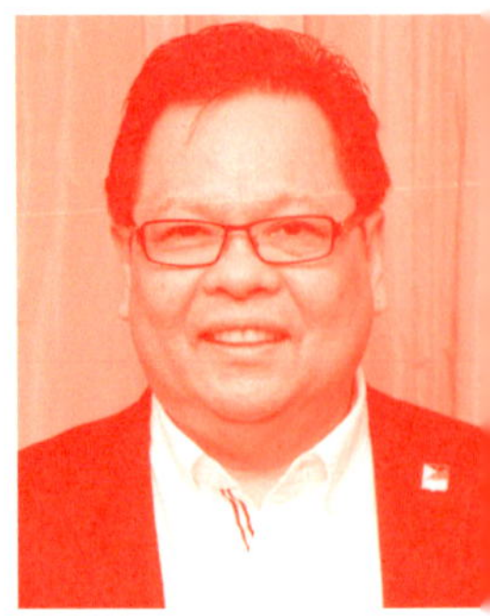
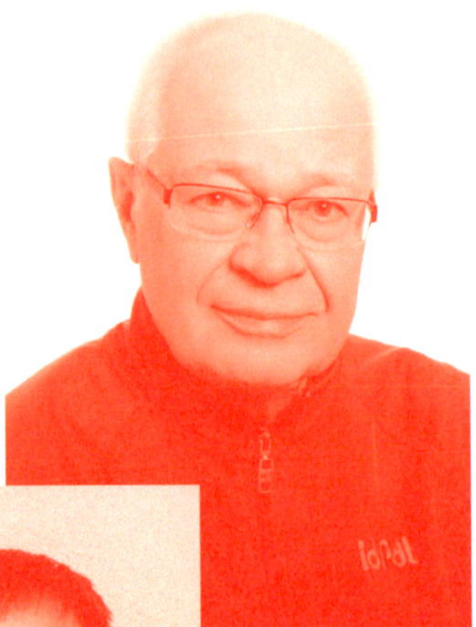
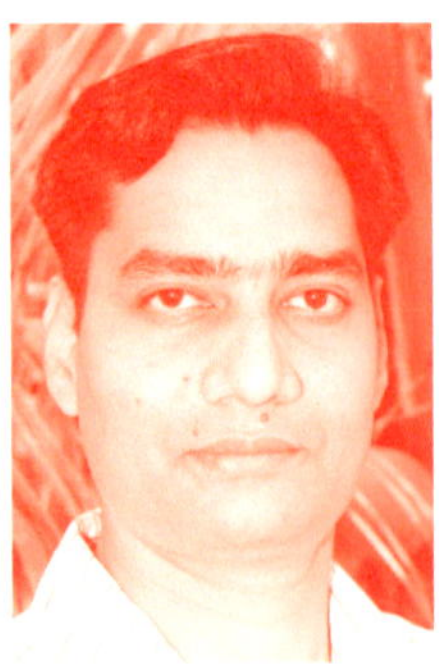
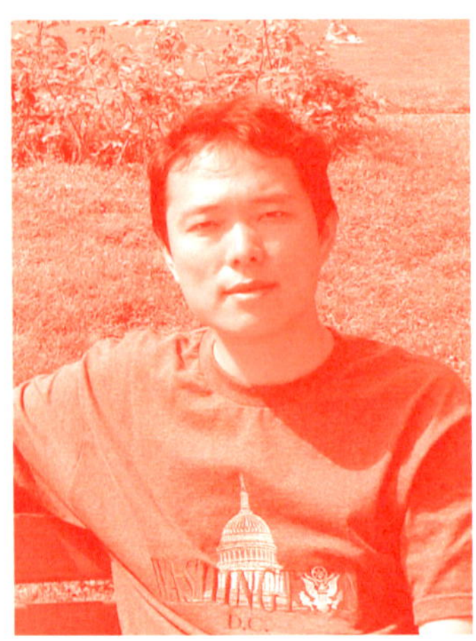
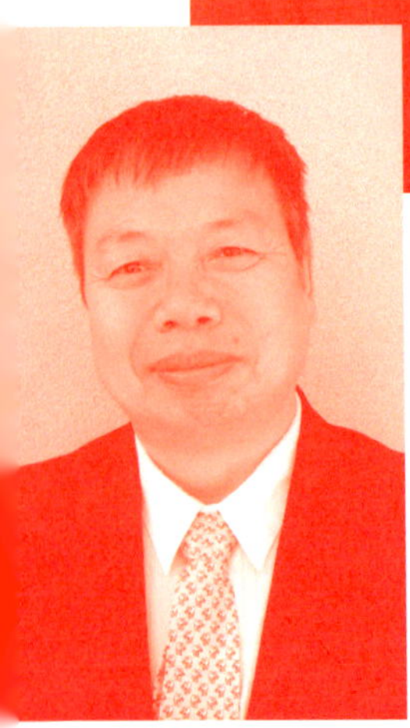
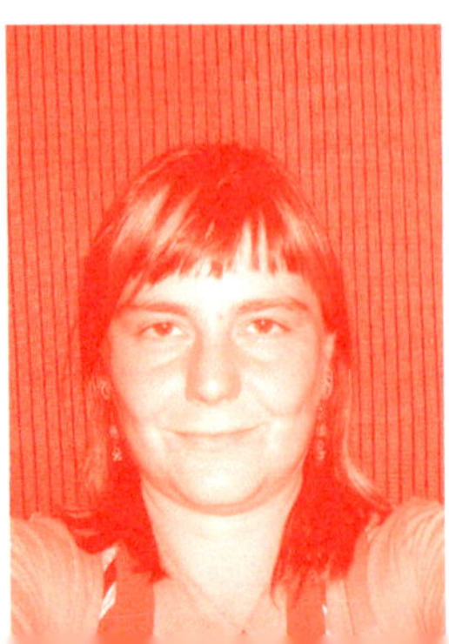

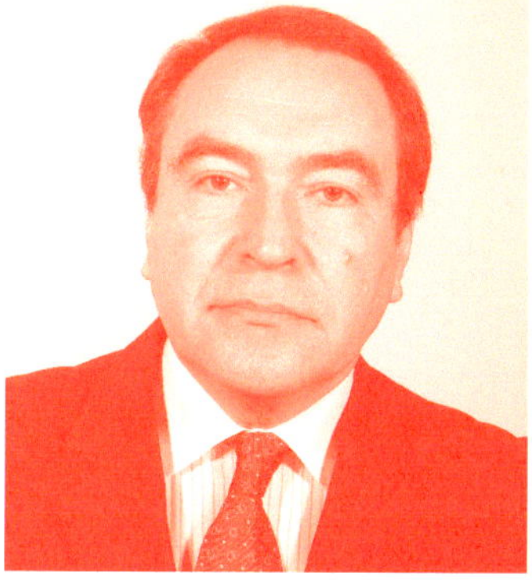
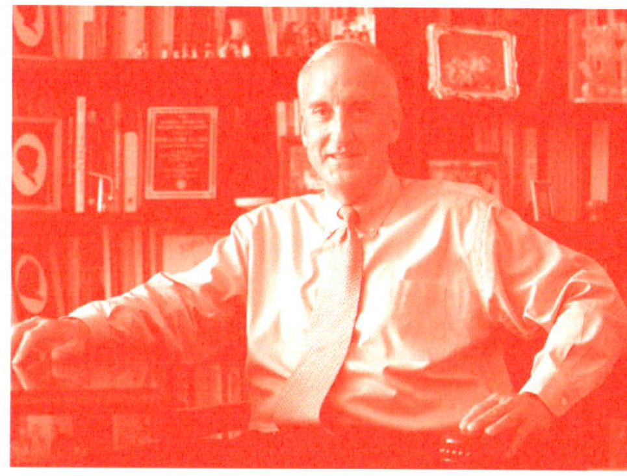
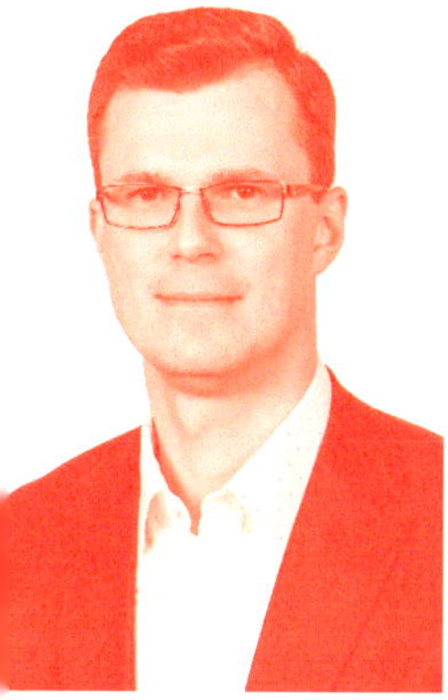
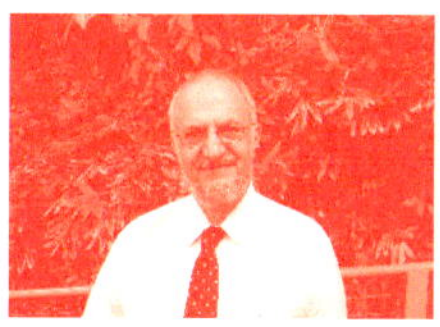
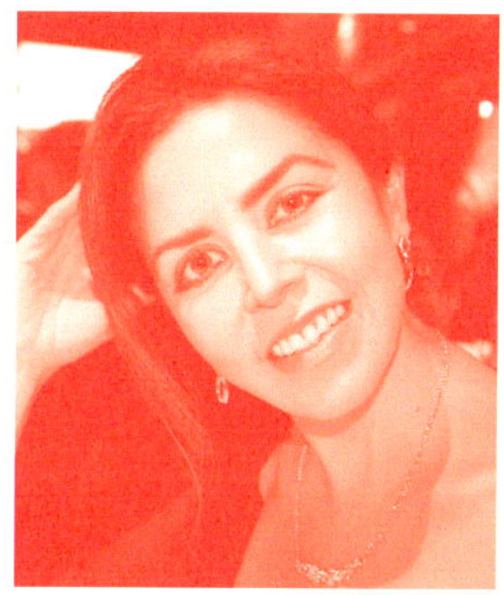

Supporting open minds since 2005

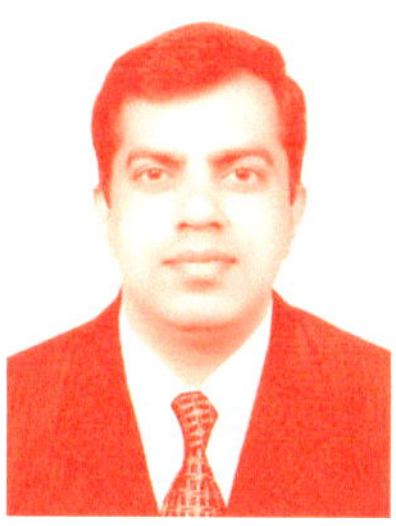
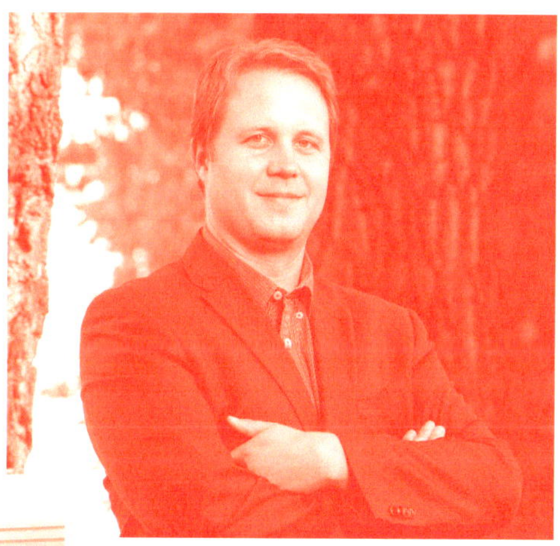
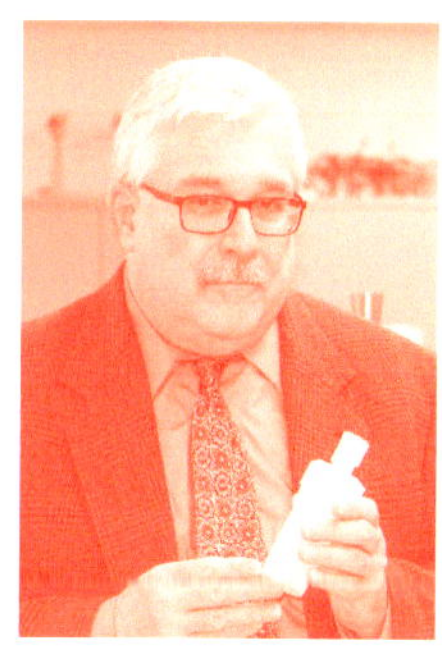
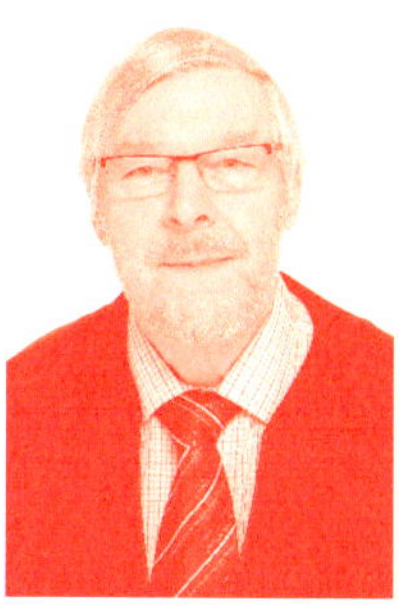
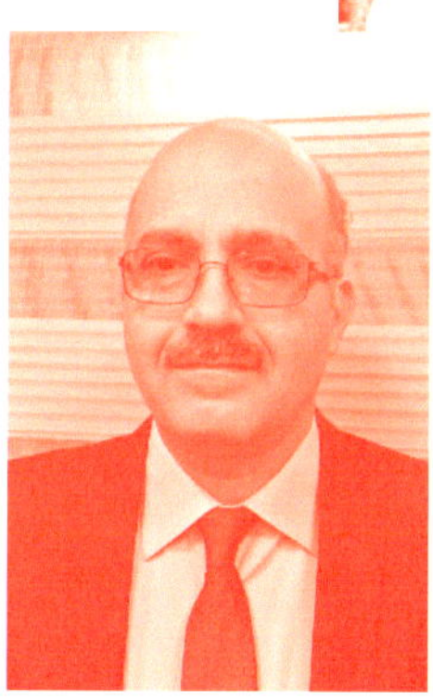
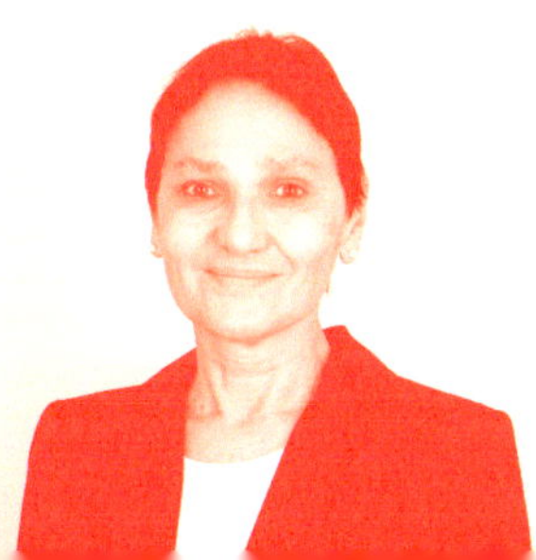
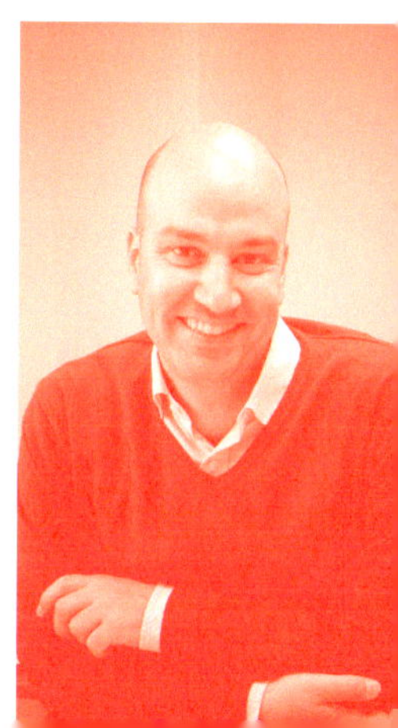

Heart Valve Surgery
http://dx.doi.org/10.5772/intechopen.94679
Edited by Sameh M. Said and Jeffrey Shuhaiber

Contributors
Anze Djordjevic, Igor Knez, Fevzi Sarper Türker, Zeki Temiztürk, Davut Azboy, Habib Rehman Khan, Muhtashim Mian, Yasuhiro Shudo, Sameh M. Said

First published in London, United Kingdom, 2022 by IntechOpen
IntechOpen is the global imprint of INTECHOPEN LIMITED, registered in England and Wales, registration number: 11086078, 5 Princes Gate Court, London, SW7 2QJ, United Kingdom
Printed in Croatia

British Library Cataloguing-in-Publication Data
A catalogue record for this book is available from the British Library

Additional hard and PDF copies can be obtained from orders@intechopen.com

Heart Valve Surgery
Edited by Sameh M. Said and Jeffrey Shuhaiber
p. cm.
Print ISBN 978-1-83969-400-4
Online ISBN 978-1-83969-401-1
eBook (PDF) ISBN 978-1-83969-402-8

For EU product safety concerns:
IN TECH d.o.o., Prolaz Marije Krucifikse Kozulić 3, 51000 Rijeka, Croatia, info@intechopen.com or visit our website at intechopen.com.

Meet the editors

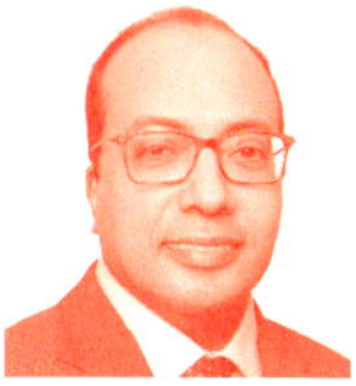

Dr. Sameh M. Said is a pediatric and adult congenital cardiac surgeon and the current chief of the Division of Pediatric and Adult Congenital Cardiac Surgery, at Maria Fareri Children's Hospital, Westchester Medical Center Health Network, USA. He previously worked as a pediatric and adult cardiac surgeon at the Mayo Clinic, USA and the University of Minnesota, USA. Dr. Said graduated from Alexandria University, Egypt, in 1998, where he also completed his cardiothoracic surgical residency. This was followed by an advanced cardiovascular surgery fellowship at Mayo Clinic, where he also completed an integrated general and thoracic surgery residency. He also completed an accredited pediatric congenital cardiac surgery fellowship at Lucile Packard's Children's Hospital, USA. Dr. Said is board certified in general, thoracic, and pediatric cardiac surgery and has special expertise and interest in neonatal surgery, complex cardiac reoperation, unifocalization and pulmonary artery branch rehabilitation, Ebstein's anomaly, hypertrophic cardiomyopathy, and the Ross procedure. He has co-authored more than 200 peer-reviewed publications and 24 book chapters and edited two books. He is an active member of many cardiothoracic surgical societies and associations.

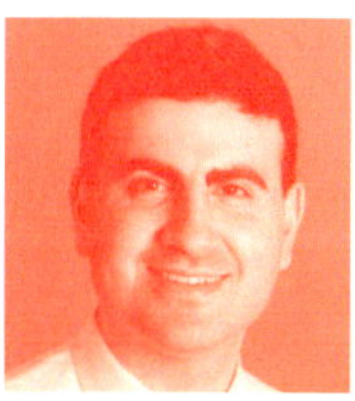

Dr. Jeffrey Shuhaiber is an adult cardiac surgeon with broad training and experience in congenital heart surgery, heart failure, and valve surgery. He is a cardiovascular surgeon practicing at the Geisinger Clinic, USA. He also is a physician investigator running a translational lab at Massachusetts General Hospital, Harvard Medical School, USA. He graduated with distinction in pharmacology and medicine from Kings College London in 1998. He completed postgraduate training in London, Chicago, Cleveland, and Boston. Dr. Shuhaiber is board certified in general surgery and thoracic surgery. He has more than eighty peer-reviewed publications and several book chapters to his credit. He has also edited three books. While focusing on surgery, he works on standardizing safety, procedures, and processes in patient care. Dr. Shuhaiber is an active member of the Society of Thoracic Surgery.

Contents

Preface

In 1952, Charles Hufnagel implanted the first artificial valve in a 30-year-old woman with severe aortic valve regurgitation. This was done in an era when open heart surgery and valve surgery did not exist, albeit there were primitive attempts to treat heart diseases at that time. Valve surgery has come a long way since then and the progress being made in treating different valve pathology today is beyond imagination.

This book highlights some of the major milestones in valve surgery. It begins with a brief introductory chapter that gives an overview of the major milestones in valve surgery, such as the increased focus on valve repair rather than replacement and the advent of minimally invasive or minimal access approaches to valve surgery. It also discusses major advances in transcatheter therapy, which is an integral part of valve disease management and can be used in all heart valves either as a primary or repeat intervention.

Chapter 2 reviews minimally invasive approaches to aortic valve disease and Chapter 3 discusses the different surgical options for pulmonary valve pathology. The tricuspid valve is no longer considered the "forgotten valve" and surgeons have changed their approach and moved towards more aggressive repair strategies for the tricuspid valve, especially when data continues to show increased morbidity and mortality for patients with tricuspid valve regurgitation on long-term follow-up. This is highlighted in Chapter 4. Chapter 5 describes the conduction system and its risk of involvement when performing different types of procedures on different heart valves. Finally, Chapter 6 examines the role of concomitant valve surgery during orthotopic heart transplantation. This is a unique situation with a unique solution to avoid repeat interventions after heart transplantation to optimize the hemodynamics of the new heart.

I am very grateful to all the contributing authors for their excellent chapters, as well as the editorial staff at IntechOpen. I also would like to thank my co-editor Dr. Jeffrey Shuhaiber for his valuable assistance in editing this book.

Sameh M. Said, MBBCh, MD, FACC, FACS
Chief,
Division of Pediatric and Adult Congenital Cardiac Surgery,
Maria Fareri Children's Hospital,
Westchester Medical Center,
Valhalla, New York, USA

Jeffrey Shuhaiber, BSc MD MBA
Cardiovascular Surgeon,
Geisinger Heart Institute,
Wilkes Barre, PA, USA

Section 1

Introduction

Chapter 1

Introductory Chapter: Heart Valve Surgery – Current Status and Future Directions

Sameh M. Said

1. Introduction

This year marks the 70th anniversary of the first artificial heart valve [1] that was implanted in 1952 by Charles Hufnagel to treat a 30-year-old woman with severe aortic regurgitation [2] in an era where the concept of direct valve repair or replacement did not exist. It is remarkable, how far we have come since then in terms of managing heart valve disease. This is not only in terms of advances in surgical techniques or choice of prostheses for different valve pathology but also in terms of transcatheter therapy and minimally invasive surgical approaches. In the current chapter, we will review briefly, the major milestones in management of different valve pathology in regard to approaches, techniques, and future directions.

2. Aortic valve

2.1 Aortic valve repair

If the aortic valve can be repaired, there is no doubt, this is the number one option for patients. This achieves the best quality of life and freedom from anticoagulation. However, the process of reconstructing the aortic valve is relatively new and is more complex in comparison to the mitral valve, which has much more robust and longer-term data in terms of durability and survival.

Aortic valve repair remains challenging and requires higher level of experience and judgment [3]. Surgeons started to pay attention in the current era to the importance of repairing the native aortic valve, and with the current trend of expansion for the valve-sparing surgery and aortic valve repair, the future of aortic valve surgery is promising.

2.2 Aortic valve replacement

2.2.1 Transcatheter valve therapy

Since the introduction of transcatheter aortic valve replacement (TAVR), and the emergence of early favorable results from the TAVR trials showing equivalent mortality and short-term survival to surgical aortic valve replacement (SAVR) [4], this form of therapy has spread widely across the globe. The procedure is no longer limited to transfemoral or transapical access as initially started, but it expanded to include other alternate accesses such as trans-carotid [5], trans-caval [6], and trans-subclavian [7]. This allows providing transcatheter therapy to the highest-risk population and further participated in its widespread with currently patient rarely get turned down for the procedure because of access limitations or procedural risks.

The procedure was associated with several morbidities in the beginning, particularly access-related, periprosthetic regurgitation and had higher risk of stroke and other neurological events. Many of these early problems have been resolved with improvements in the delivery system, valve design, and the use of cerebral protection devices [8]. One other major advance is the ability to perform these procedures without general anesthesia and in a totally percutaneous fashion with no incisions. This contributed markedly to rapid recovery, shorter length of hospital stay, and quicker return to activity.

TAVR did not stop at the high-risk patients and further expanded to the medium and low-risk populations. Whether this is a good strategy or not, remains to be determined.

2.2.2 Choice of the surgical prosthesis

With the expansion of transcatheter valve therapy, it-without doubt-changed the choice of the prosthesis, even in younger patients with more and more tendency to using bioprostheses, despite knowing the need for repeat operation or repeat interventions.

While the data remains in favor of implanting mechanical prostheses in young patients in terms of survival [9], this did not result in its expansion, and bioprosthesis continues to be number one prosthetic implant in the current era. The On-X® prosthesis (Cryolife Inc., Kennesaw, GA, USA) was utilized on a widescale recently with the goal to use a lower anticoagulation target and may be avoiding standard anticoagulation to provide both a better quality of life and the best durability. The result of the PROACT trial was quite disappointing when the data showed higher risk of adverse events in patients receiving apixaban, and the trial was stopped [10].

Developing a new prosthetic design that is durable and requires low or no anticoagulation will be a key that may change the paradigm in the future in regard to the choice of the valve prosthesis.

2.2.3 Aortic annular enlargement

Recent data showed that there was a trend of placing small aortic prostheses in the previous era, which resulted in higher number of patients experiencing patient-prosthesis mismatch, and need for repeat operations.

With the expansion of transcatheter therapy, data shows that implanting transcatheter valves inside degenerated smaller-size prostheses will result in creating gradient across that left ventricular outflow tract [11]. More emerging data supportive of the negative impact of patient-prosthesis mismatch on survival [12] drew the attention of the surgical community and currently, there are more trends to enlarge the aortic annulus with a variety of surgical techniques to accommodate a large enough prosthesis that will facilitate future transcatheter therapy.

2.2.4 Advances in minimally invasive approaches

With the advent of transcatheter therapy and the obvious advantage of minimal to no incisions needed and the quick return to activities, this stimulated the surgical community to think of alternative accesses to aortic valve repair or replacement. A variety has been pioneered by several centers and expands from robotic [13], to totally endoscopic [14], to minimally invasive right axillary thoracotomy or anterior thoracotomy [15] and upper mini-sternotomy.

While most data do not show major differences between upper sternotomy and right anterior mini-thoracotomy in terms of 30-day mortality [16], it is to be determined, the longer-term data of other minimally invasive approaches in comparison to standard sternotomy.

2.2.5 Ross renaissance

Ross procedure continues to cause debate over the years, however, with more recent and robust data coming out of several institutions across the globe, there has been an upward trend in utilization of the Ross procedure, especially in young adults. Data shows better long-term survival and excellent quality of life in young adults after the Ross procedure [17]. This makes the procedure currently the number one of choice as a replacement option in young adults and those who have an active lifestyle and do not want anticoagulation.

It remains to be determined if this trend will continue especially in the continuing expansion of transcatheter therapy and the technical challenges that are needed for the Ross operation or its repeat interventions.

3. Mitral valve

The progress in mitral valve surgery has been in parallel with aortic valve surgery in terms of the expansion of the minimally invasive approaches and the importance of repairing the valve whenever possible. The choice of the surgical prosthesis has been shifted in a similar manner to the aortic valve with more tendency for bioprosthesis and lower trend for the mechanical ones.

Recently, transcatheter therapy has progressed from being an initial option for degenerated mitral prostheses (valve-in-valve) and recurrent valvular regurgitation (valve-in-ring) to primary interventions in native mitral valve disease. This role of transcatheter therapy has been growing to involve edge-to-edge repair and mitral valve replacement in calcified mitral annulus. Long-term data are needed to determine the appropriate application of these transcatheter therapies.

4. Tricuspid valve

Tricuspid valve has been known for a long-time as the "forgotten valve" as there was a tendency not to address tricuspid valve regurgitation, especially in the settings of left-sided pathology. A misconception that tricuspid regurgitation will improve once the left-sided lesions are addressed, however, time has proven that this is inaccurate and tricuspid regurgitation should be treated at the time of the initial heart surgery. An upward trend that we started to see in the current era due to the negative long-term effects of significant tricuspid regurgitation on survival.

This even expanded to offer tricuspid valve annuloplasty in absence of tricuspid regurgitation but in the presence of the annular dilation to prevent adverse remodeling of the right ventricle and the development of future significant regurgitation [18].

Recently, transcatheter therapy started to play a role in tricuspid valve disease, especially in high-risk patients *via* application of edge-to-edge repair in a similar fashion to the mitral valve or bicaval valve implantation [19] or standard transcatheter valve implantation [20]. Long-term data will be needed to prove the efficacy of these techniques.

5. Future directions

No doubt the current era has witnessed major milestones in both the transcatheter and surgical aspects of valve therapy. This, while provides several options to patients with every valve disease, it also creates confusion on which is the better option. This demonstrates the importance of having a heart valve team with all the expertise available for surgical, both open and minimally invasive, and transcatheter therapy. This should provide the patients and their families with unbiased opinions that suites each individual patient and give them the best option that is good for their expected survival, and desired quality of life and matches their future expectations.

Disclosures

The author S.M.S. is a consultant to Artivion, Abbott, and Stryker.

Author details

Sameh M. Said[1,2]

1 Division of Pediatric and Adult Congenital Cardiac Surgery, Maria Fareri Children's Hospital, Department of Surgery, Westchester Medical Center, Valhalla, New York, USA

2 Faculty of Medicine, Department of Cardiothoracic Surgery, Alexandria University, Alexandria, Egypt

*Address all correspondence to: sameh.said@wmchealth.org

References

[1] Said SM. The 70th anniversary of the first artificial heart valve "from a plastic valve to homotransplantation to cusp type valves". Journal of Cardiac Surgery. Dec 2022;**37**(12):5670-5680

[2] Hufnagel CA, Conrad PW. The direct approach for the correction of aortic insufficiency. Journal of the American Medical Association. 1961;**178**(3):275-279

[3] Aazami M, Schäfers H-J. Advances in heart valve surgery. Journal of Interventional Cardiology. 2003;**16**(6):535-541

[4] Hamm CW, Arsalan M, Mack MJ. The future of transcatheter aortic valve implantation. European Heart Journal. 2015;**6**:8644

[5] Overtchouk P, Folliguet T, Pinaud F, et al. Transcarotid approach for transcatheter aortic valve replacement with the Sapien 3 prosthesis: A multicenter french registry. JACC: Cardiovascular Interventions. 2019;**12**(5):413-419

[6] Muhammad K, Tokarchik GC. Transcaval transcatheter aortic valve replacement: A visual case review. Journal of Visualized Surgery. 2018;**4**:102

[7] Kasapkara HA, Aslan AN, Ayhan H, et al. Trans-subclavian aortic valve replacement with various bioprosthetic valves: Single-center experience. Türk Kardiyoloji Derneği Arşivi. 2016;**44**(7):582-589

[8] Stachon P, Kaier K, Heidt T, et al. The use and outcomes of cerebral protection devices for patients undergoing transfemoral transcatheter aortic valve replacement in clinical practice. JACC: Cardiovascular Interventions. 2021;**14**(2):161-168

[9] Badhwar V, Ofenloch JC, Rovin JD, van Gelder HM, Jacobs JP. Noninferiority of closely monitored mechanical valves to bioprostheses overshadowed by early mortality benefit in younger patients. The Annals of Thoracic Surgery. 2012;**93**:748-753

[10] Artivion Inc. Artivion follows recommendation to stop PROACT Xa clinical trial – Artivion, Inc., at 7:00 AM EDT. 23 September 2022. [Accessed: December 20, 2022]

[11] Alnajar A, Hamad N, Azhar MZ, Mousa Y, Arora Y, Lamelas J. Surgical versus transcatheter aortic valve replacement: Impact of patient-prosthesis mismatch on outcomes. Journal of Cardiac Surgery. Dec 2022;**37**(12):5388-5394

[12] Head SJ, Mokhles MM, Osnabrugge RL, et al. The impact of prosthesis-patient mismatch on long-term survival after aortic valve replacement: A systematic review and meta-analysis of 34 observational studies comprising 27 186 patients with 133 141 patient-years. European Heart Journal. Dec 2012;**37**(12):5388-5394

[13] Tamadon I, Soldani G, Dario P, Menciassi A. Novel robotic approach for minimally invasive aortic heart valve surgery. Annu Int Conf IEEE Eng Med Biol Soc. 2018 Jul; 2018. pp. 3656-3659

[14] Yilmaz A, Van Genechten S, Claessens J, Packlé L, Maessen J, Kaya A. A totally endoscopic approach for aortic valve surgery. European Journal of Cardio-Thoracic Surgery. 2022;**62**(6):ezac 467

[15] Ramchandani MK, Wyler von Ballmoos MC, Reardon MJ. Minimally invasive surgical aortic valve replacement through a right anterior

thoracotomy: How I teach it. The Annals of Thoracic Surgery. 2019;**107**(1):19-23

[16] Bakhtiary F, Salamate S, Amer M, Sirat S, Bayram A, Doss M, et al. Comparison of right anterior mini-thoracotomy versus partial upper sternotomy in aortic valve replacement. Advances in Therapy. 2022;**39**(9): 4266-4284

[17] Kalfa D, Mohammadi S, Kalavrouziotis D, et al. Long-term outcomes of the Ross procedure in adults with severe aortic stenosis: Single-centre experience with 20 years of follow-up. European Journal of Cardio-Thoracic Surgery. 2015;**47**(1): 159-167

[18] Dietz MF, van Wijngaarden AL, Mack MJ, et al. Long-term impact of preventive tricuspid valve annuloplasty on right ventricular remodeling. The American Journal of Cardiology. 2022;**169**:93-99

[19] Jin QW, Ghazi ABM, Kolanthaivelu J, Yahaya SA. Novel treatment of atrial functional tricuspid regurgitation using transcatheter bicaval valve implantation (TricValve). Asia Intervention. 2022;**8**(2):138-142

[20] Kang Z, Shi J, Liu L, Guo Y. Transjugular transcatheter tricuspid valve replacement for original valve regurgitation. JACC. Cardiovascular Interventions. 2022;**15**(22):2339-2340

Section 2

Aortic Valve

Chapter 2

Minimally Invasive Aortic Valve Surgery

Anze Djordjevic and Igor Knez

Abstract

Minimally invasive aortic valve surgery by definition means performing procedures through alternative approaches without the need to divide the sternum completely. Even though this contributes towards lowering the mortality and morbidity of patients, minimally invasive techniques have to be tailored to the unique patient as well as surgeon characteristics. With the advancements made in invasive cardiology techniques, the line between invasive cardiology and minimally invasive cardiac surgery is becoming thinner and thinner. We are presenting state-of-the-art techniques and outcomes for surgical aortic valve replacement via upper mini-sternotomy or anterior right mini-thoracotomy. In addition, aortic valve repair and valve-sparing procedures through a minimally invasive approach are discussed.

Keywords: aortic valve, valve surgery, minimally invasive surgery, upper mini-sternotomy, right anterior mini-thoracotomy

1. Introduction

Modern and complex aortic valve surgery is dependent on extracorporeal circulation established first in 1953 by Gibbon [1]. The first, Hufnagel's aortic valve was implanted in the descending aorta in 1956 [2] and from then on annual numbers of aortic valve procedures performed through a full median sternotomy have risen significantly over the next decades. In 2002, Cribier performed the first transcatheter aortic valve implantation (TAVI), which paved the way for percutaneously resolving patients with prohibitive surgical risk [3]. Although, first minimally invasive approaches were developed a decade earlier, they gained increased interest after ever looser indications for TAVI. That dictated a response from the cardiac surgery society. Cosgrove performed the first minimally invasive aortic valve replacement (AVR) through a right parasternal approach back in 1996 [4]. In the same decade, more minimally invasive approaches were developed, such as upper mini-sternotomy, anterior right mini-thoracotomy (ART) or transverse sternotomy. Today, most isolated AVRs are performed through either upper mini-sternotomy or ART (**Figure 1**) with reduced pain, improved respiratory function, early recovery and an overall reduction in trauma.

Regardless of the approach, some essentials must not be compromised in aortic valve surgery. These include safe application of a stable aortic cross-clamp, adequate visualization of the aortic valve, ensuring the same degree of myocardial protection as in median sternotomy, enabled approach to the aortic root and ascending aorta, and ability to quickly convert to median sternotomy if needed.

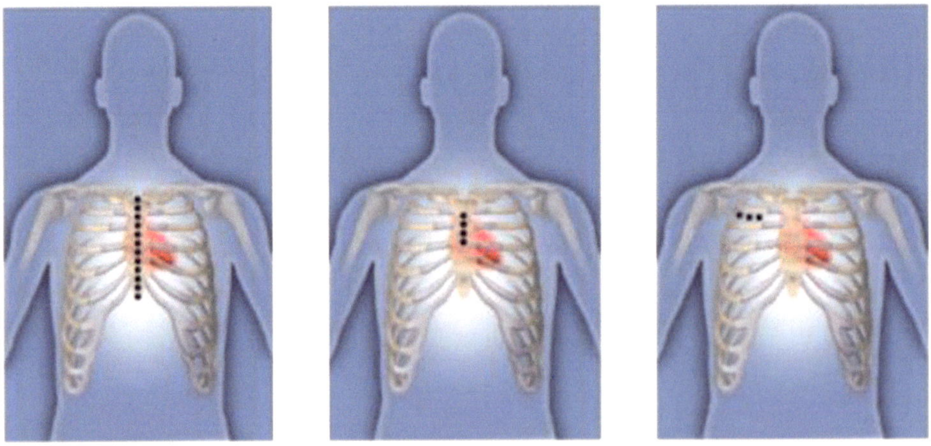

Figure 1.
Different approaches for aortic valve surgery. Left: median sternotomy; middle: upper mini-sternotomy; right: anterior right mini-thoracotomy.

The present chapter aims to describe the two most commonly used minimally invasive approaches to aortic valve surgery (upper mini-sternotomy and ART) with a special focus on surgical technique and outcomes.

2. Upper mini-sternotomy

Skin incision runs over the upper half of the sternum and is usually <10 cm long. Sternotomy can be performed with either the standard (our preference) or oscillating saw and is performed in a "J" matter into the right 3rd (Maribor preference) or 4th (Graz preference) intercostal space. The selected intercostal space is determined by the total sternal length, method of myocardial protection delivery (antegrade or combined ante–/retrograde cardioplegia) and surgeon preference. If exposure of the aortic valve is not satisfying, the "J" mini-sternotomy can be modified to a "T" mini-sternotomy or converted to a full median sternotomy. However, care must be taken during sternotomy osteosynthesis when more than two sternal fragments are present to avoid excessive postoperative bleeding or sternal dehiscence. In upper "J" mini-sternotomy, prophylactic division of the right internal thoracic artery (RITA) is not required.

A small-blade retractor is inserted and the pericardium is opened in a longitudinal matter (**Figure 2**) [5]. Two to three stay sutures on both sides are applied and the intrapericardial contents are lifted upwards. Care must be taken not to reduce cardiac preload, which could lead to patient deterioration in the presence of severe aortic valve stenosis.

The cardiopulmonary bypass could be established centrally or peripherally. At our institutions, central cannulation remains the preferred option except in cases of severe ascending aortic calcifications. After systemic heparinization with 300 I.U./kg to achieve an activated clotting time (ACT) > 480 s, the distal ascending aorta is cannulated through two Prolene 3-0 purse-string sutures with pledgets placed in a circular fashion. A double-stage venous cannula is placed through a single Prolene 3-0 purse-string suture either through the right atrial appendage (Graz preference) or in the superior vena cava (Maribor preference). When cannulating the right atrial appendage, the venous cannula could be positioned to the side of the mini-sternotomy wound or under the undivided sternum and beneath the xiphoid (**Figure 3**) [6].

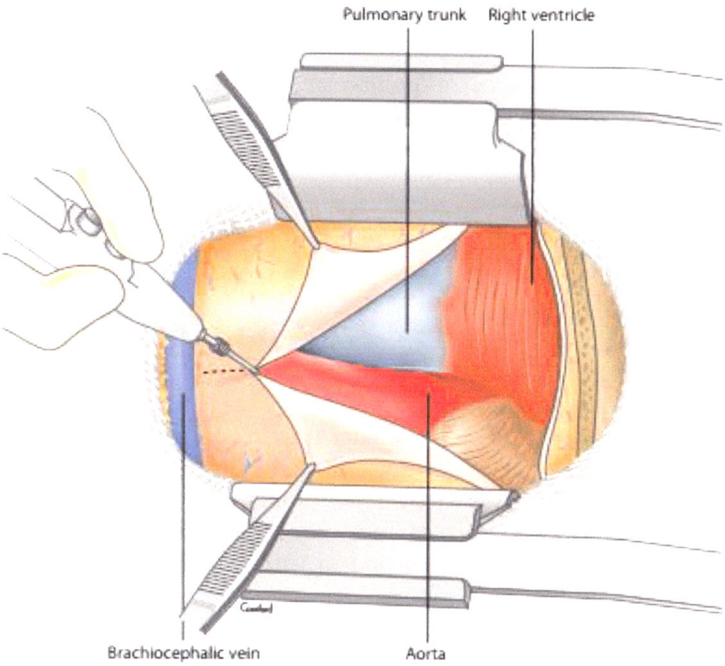

Figure 2.
Incision of the pericardium through an upper mini-sternotomy [5].

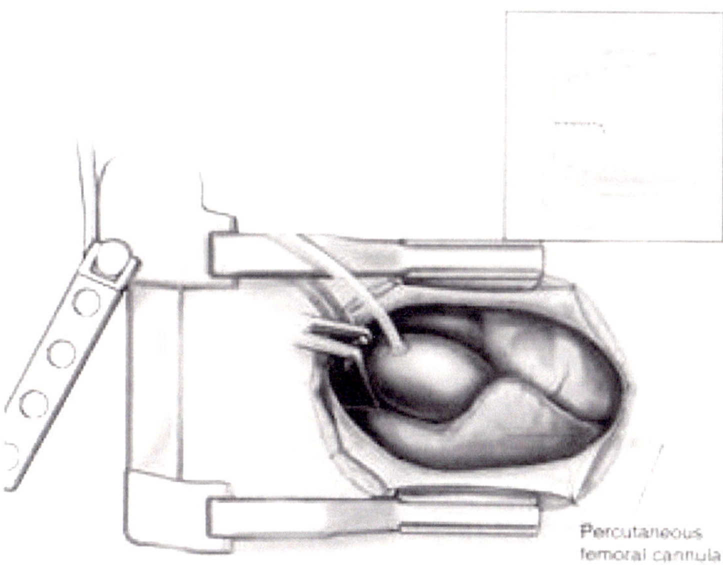

Figure 3.
Upper mini-sternotomy. Operative field and sternal incision [6].

The choice of cardioplegia dictates the type of cannulation. Some cardioplegic solutions (for example del Nido extracellular crystalloid cardioplegia) require only antegrade delivery. On the other hand, other solutions (such as blood cardioplegia or St. Thomas extracellular crystalloid cardioplegia) enhance myocardial protection when administered via both ante- and retrograde fashion. In that case, the retrograde cardioplegic cannula is inserted in the coronary sinus through a single Prolene 3-0 U-suture placed between the venous cannula and the inferior vena cava.

The antegrade cardioplegic cannula is inserted in the proximal ascending aorta through a single Prolene 3-0 U-suture.

After placing the patient on cardiopulmonary bypass, a left ventricular vent is placed through the right superior pulmonary vein or directly through the aorta. Patients could be safely operated on in normothermia (Maribor preference) or mild hypothermia (34°C) (Graz preference).

The aorta is cross-clamped, cardioplegia is administered and the intrapericardial sac is flushed with cold saline to topically cool the heart. An oblique semicircular incision is made into the ascending aorta and three stay sutures are applied to each commissure (**Figure 4**) [5].

The aortic valve is excised with a 2-mm margin-left on the aortic annulus. After flushing the left ventricular outflow tract (LVOT) and ascending aorta to remove residual calcified particles, an appropriate artificial valve sizer is introduced. Interrupted Ticron 2-0 U-sutures with pledgets are placed through the annulus with pledgets on the ventricular side. Care must be taken on the commissure between the right and a coronary leaflets not to injure the AV node. When an appropriate valve size is chosen, these sutures are placed on the sewing ring and the valve is lowered into the aortic annulus. The sutures are tied either by hand or by novel artificial tying devices (e.g., Cor-Knot). Coronary ostia are carefully inspected to prevent catastrophic consequences (**Figure 5**).

The aortotomy is closed using two Prolene 4-0 running sutures, both starting at the aortotomy edges. The patient is rewarmed if needed and the heart is de-aired mostly through a needle incision in the ascending aorta, just distal to the aortotomy. After removing the aortic cross-clamp, a rhythm check is required. If ventricular fibrillation, external defibrillation is applied. When sinus rhythm occurs, an epicardial temporary pacemaker wire is placed on the right ventricle. This maneuver is facilitated when the heart is actively emptied through the venous cannula and the wire is then pulled out through the 3rd right intercostal space.

Also, during active venous drainage, the external drains are placed. Usually, one retrosternal drain is sufficient placed either through the subxiphoid area or

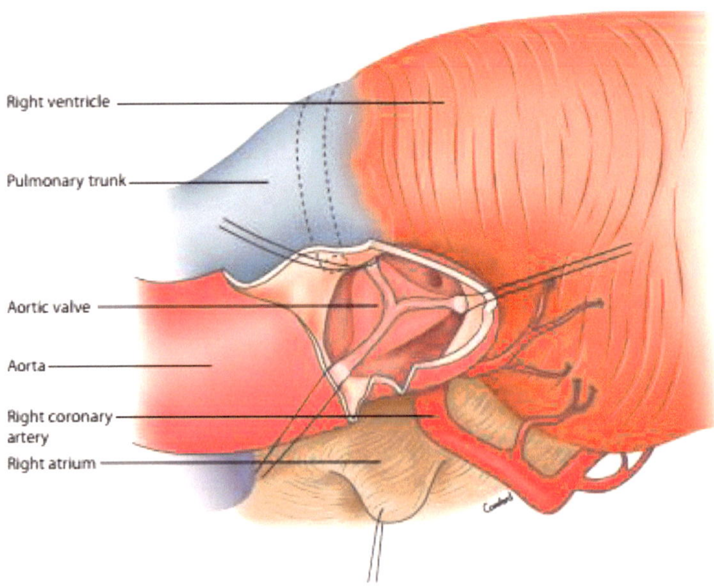

Figure 4.
Superior view of the aortic valve [5].

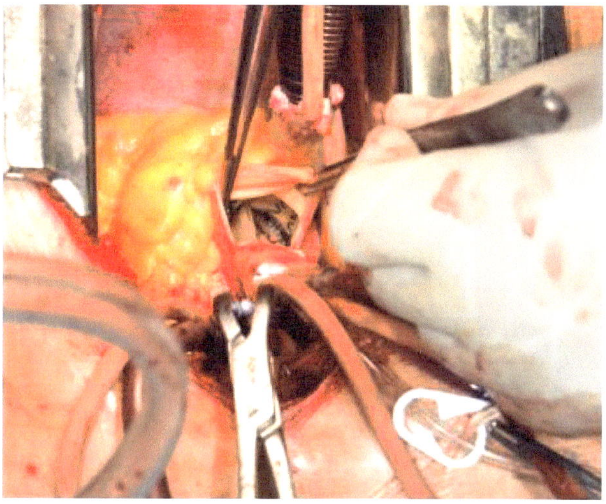

Figure 5.
Probing the coronary ostia (courtesy of Medical University of Graz).

the 3rd right intercostal space lateral to the RITA. Another viable option is also placement of transpleural drainage tubes.

Weaning from cardiopulmonary bypass follows after complete reperfusion with step-by-step decannulation and oversewing all cannulated spots with Prolene 5-0. Simultaneously with aortic decannulation, protamine is administered in a 1:1 ratio to reverse the effects of heparine. With the pericardium left open, sternal osteosynthesis is performed with one obliquely placed wire between the non-divided lower sternum and the 2nd right intercostal space and one figure-of-eight placed wire around the manubrio-sternal joint. Finally, fascia, subcutaneous tissue and skin are sutured, respectively.

3. Anterior right mini-thoracotomy

To consider this approach, a preoperative chest computed tomography (CT) scan is mandatory to assess the relationship of intrathoracic structures, especially the distance of the aortic root to the right-sided rib cage. The main criteria are: (1) the position of more than half of the ascending aorta is over the pulmonary artery on the right side of the sternum and (2) the distance of the ascending aorta from the sternum is <10 cm [7, 8]. Over the 2nd right intercostal space, a <10 cm long incision is made with the medial portion at the sternal edge. The intercostal muscles are sharply divided using electrocautery. Upon entering the thoracic cavity, the superior right pulmonary lobe is retracted using selective bilateral lung intubation and prophylactic division of the RITA is necessary to prevent extensive blood loss. A small-blade retractor is inserted and the pericardium is opened in a longitudinal matter (**Figure 6**) [5]. It is of paramount importance to identify the phrenic nerve before pericardial incision to avoid postoperative delayed mechanical ventilation due to respiratory disturbances. Two stay sutures on both sides are applied and the intrapericardial contents are lifted upwards. We advise against routine rib resection. In most ART cases, visualization is already satisfactory after intercostal muscles' division.

The cardiopulmonary bypass could be established centrally or peripherally. At our institutions, central cannulation remains the preferred option. The rest of the operation commences in a similar fashion as previously described in the chapter on upper mini-sternotomy [9, 10].

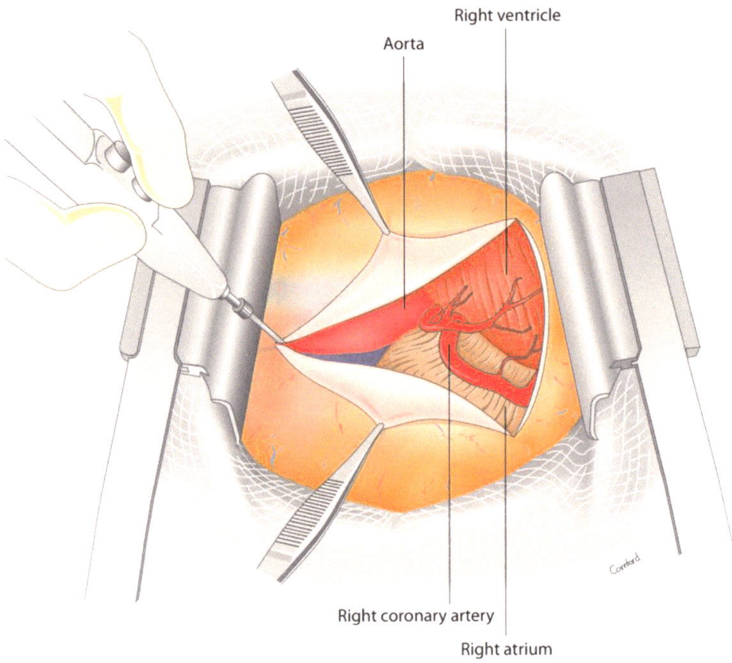

Figure 6.
Pericardial incision through an anterior right mini-thoracotomy [5].

4. Outcomes

Both already described minimally invasive approaches to the aortic valve were developed in the 1990s. The Cleveland group developed the upper mini-sternotomy technique in 1996 [4] and the first published data on the ART are from New Delhi group from 1993 [9].

The first large published article regarding minimally invasive aortic valve surgery was written by the Boston group. They reported their experience with 526 consecutive minimally invasive aortic valve procedures, which were mostly done through an upper mini-sternotomy (93%). Their publication has shown excellent results with short- and long-term mortality at 2% and 5%, respectively. Freedom from reoperation at 6 years was 99% [6].

Encouraged by these data, the number of minimally invasive aortic valve surgery have risen significantly in the following years. A report was recently published on the clinical trends between median sternotomy and minimally invasive approaches for aortic valve stenosis in three high volume aortic valve surgery centres in the USA (Houston, Atlanta, and Miami). In the observed three-year period, the overall number of AVRs increased by 107% owing to improved diagnostics and TAVIs for previously denied patients. Minimally invasive AVRs increased by 57% and median sternotomy AVRs decreased by 15% [11].

Outcomes of minimally invasive aortic valve surgery are similar or even superior in some reports to those of conventional median sternotomy surgery [12].

4.1 Mortality

Mortality rates are similar when comparing ART [13–15] or upper mini-sternotomy [6, 16, 17] with median sternotomy, respectively. One-year survival is reported to be >95%, whereas 5-year survival ranges from 80–95%, respectively.

4.2 Postoperative bleeding

The incidence of re-exploration due to excessive bleeding ranges from 3.8% up to 12% [15–18]. The latter high number was reported by Semsroth et al. in a subgroup of 167 patients who were operated through an ART. One explanation could be that they already experienced lots of issues with intraoperative bleeding, which resulted in the fact that bleeding was the predominant cause for conversion to median sternotomy [18]. Most often significant bleeding occurs on the aortotomy edges, on cannulation sites, especially the right superior pulmonary vein, on sternotomy edges or if the RITA is injured.

4.3 Transfusion

Blood product transfusion is reported to be significantly lower in minimally invasive aortic valve surgery compared to traditional median sternotomy. Reported incidences are from 21.3% to 48.8% [13–18]. The highest reported incidence was by Stolinski et al. in a series of 211 patients who undergone an ART, which is still significantly lower than in the median sternotomy group (67.3%, $p < 0.001$) [15].

4.4 Postoperative atrial fibrillation

Rhythm disturbances often accompany cardiac valvular procedures. The reported incidences of postoperative atrial fibrillation (POAF) are from 12.8% to 32.2% [13, 15–17].

4.5 Mechanical ventilation

Mechanical ventilation is significantly shorter in patients undergoing minimally invasive aortic valve surgery (5 vs. 6 h; $p = 0.04$) [17] and only 4.3% required prolonged ventilation >24 h [16].

4.6 Intensive care unit and hospital stay

Intensive care unit (ICU) and hospital length of stay are perhaps the most evident advantages of minimally invasive aortic valve surgery. Both parameters are shorter in comparison to median sternotomy aortic valve surgery [15]. Semsroth et al. reported a mean duration of ICU to stay 22 h for upper mini-sternotomy and 21 h for ART patients [18]. Although, Ghanta et al. reported longer ICU stays, early discharge defined by discharge by the 4th postoperative day (POD) was achieved in 15.8% in the minimally invasive group compared to only 4.2% in the median sternotomy group ($p < 0.01$) [17]. About 52.8% of minimally invasive surgery patients are discharged by the 6th POD and only 7.9% have a prolonged stay over 12 days [16].

4.7 Acute kidney injury

Acute kidney injury (AKI) incidence ranges from 1% to 4.7% [16, 17] with hemodialysis from 0.5% to 13.2% [15, 18]. The large differences are a consequence of different AKI definitions and acquired protocols for renal replacement therapy. The highest reported incidence of hemodialysis comes from the report by Semsroth et al. Their explanation lies in the necessity of a preoperative CT imaging for patients receiving minimally invasive aortic valve surgery through ART, as contrast enhancement is nephrotoxic and might increase the risk for AKI [18].

However, a word of caution is proper. Not all patients are suitable for minimally invasive approaches, especially for ART which is technically more demanding. The reported exclusion criteria for ART are concomitant ascending aortic aneurysms, ascending aorta located completely retrosternal or relatively left lateral, pathological calcification of the ascending aorta (soft plaques) or prior cardiac surgery, history of right-sided pleuritis, a deep chest or women with large breasts [10, 19]. On the other hand, this approach is highly beneficial for disabled patients on crutches or those with deformed sternum due to radiation or injury.

5. Aortic valve repair and valve-sparing procedures through a minimally invasive approach

All of the information on minimally invasive approaches so far have been regarding AVR. In recent years, some authors have published their experience with performing aortic valve repair or aortic valve-sparing procedures through minimally invasive approaches.

The Beijing group reported their results in upper mini-sternotomy aortic root surgery. A relatively small sample of 18 patients was matched with an equally large median sternotomy group. There were no differences in the categories of surgery, as aortic root surgery was combined with ascending aorta replacement or aortic arch replacement. Aortic cross-clamp was significantly longer in the minimally invasive group. Regarding postoperative outcomes, fewer transfusions, lower drainage volume, shorter mechanical ventilation time as well as shorter ICU and hospital stay were observed [20].

The ART approach was tested for the treatment of ascending aortic pathology. The Houston group compared 74 patients who operated through an ART with 103 patients with median sternotomy. In a matched cohort, a trend towards longer aortic cross-clamp time as well as significantly higher numbers of the bicuspid aortic valves in the ART group was observed. Again, fewer transfusions, shorter ventilation time, shorter ICU and hospital stay were experienced. Interestingly, short-term mortality was similar between the two groups [21].

A systematic review of the results of the minimally invasive aortic root, ascending aorta or aortic arch performed by the Bristol group revealed similar mortality, decreased length of cardiopulmonary bypass, shorter ICU and hospital stay, fewer reoperations due to bleeding and lower incidence of postoperative AKI in the minimally invasive group. A major limitation of this review is very low-quality non-randomized evidence [22].

The Warsaw group reported their experience with 167 upper mini-sternotomy aortic root or ascending aorta operations. About 49% undergone ascending aortic replacement, 26% a combination of ascending aortic and aortic valve replacement and 25% one of the aortic valve-sparing procedure (reimplantation/remodeling). Short- and long-term mortality was 1% and 5%, respectively. Seven % reoperations for bleeding, 1.7% prolonged ICU stays and 4.8% postoperative AKIs were observed [23].

6. Pitfalls in minimally invasive surgery

As already mentioned in the text above, there are some specific pitfalls encountered in minimally invasive aortic valve surgery. Let us summarize and emphasize the most frequently seen:

- injury to the RITA (prophylactic division is recommended in ART, sharp tissue division and electrocautery use should prevent RITA injury in upper mini-sternotomy),
- poor exposure (excision of the prepericardial fatty tissue),
- difficult ascending aortic cannulation (always be prepared for peripheral cannulation, most often through the femoral artery),
- difficult de-airing (using a gauze-covered long instrument and additional CO_2 inflation during the procedure can help aid against air embolisms),
- reoperation (we strongly advocate against using minimally invasive approaches for redo surgery),
- do not jeopardize the patient's safety—if severe difficulties occur during a minimally invasive approach, do not hesitate to convert it into full median sternotomy.

7. Conclusions

Minimally invasive aortic valve surgery carries substantial benefits to patients with aortic valve disease. Fewer transfusions, shorter ICU and hospital stay, shorter mechanical ventilation alongside similar survival, POAF and AKI incidence are the main advantages when compared to conventional median sternotomy. The cardiac surgery society should aim at providing additional training to all cardiac surgeons to implement minimally invasive approaches in the majority of patients. Only by doing so, the cardiac surgery society can offer a counter-balance to ever-increasing numbers of TAVI, which will undoubtedly spread also in moderate or even low-risk patients in the following years [24].

Acknowledgements

The authors report not received funding.

Conflict of interest

The authors report no conflicts of interest.

Author details

Anze Djordjevic[1]* and Igor Knez[2]

1 Department of Cardiac Surgery, University Medical Center Maribor, Maribor, Slovenia

2 Department of Cardiac Surgery, Medical University of Graz, Graz, Austria

*Address all correspondence to: anze.djordjevic@ukc-mb.si; anze.djordjevic@gmail.com

References

[1] Gibbon JH. Application of a mechanical heart and lung apparatus to cardiac surgery. Minnesota medicine. 1954;**37**(3):171-185

[2] Dhillon BS, Fawcett AW. Treatment of aortic insufficiency by the Hufnagel valve with four illustrative cases. Postgraduate Medical Journal. 1956; **32**(371):438-443

[3] Cribier A, Eltchaninoff H, Bash A, et al. Percutaneous transcatheter implantation of an aortic valve prosthesis for calcific aortic stenosis: First human case description. Circulation. 2002;**106**(24):3006-3008

[4] Cosgrove DM, Sabik JF. Minimally invasive approach for aortic valve operations. The Annals of Thoracic Surgery. 1996;**62**(2):596-597

[5] Berdajs D, Turina M. Operative Anatomy of the Heart. 1st ed. Berlin: Springer-Verlag; 2011. p. 543. DOI: 10.1007/978-3-540-69229-4

[6] Mihaljevic T, Cohn LH, Unic D, et al. One thousand minimally invasive valve operations: Early and late results. Annals of Surgery. 2004;**240**(3): 529-534

[7] Glauber M, Ferrarini M, Miceli A. Minimally invasive aortic valve surgery: State of the art and future directions. Annals of Cardiothoracic Surgery. 2015;**4**(1):26-32

[8] Malaisrie SC, Barnhart GR, Farivar RS, et al. Current era minimally invasive aortic valve replacement: Techniques and practice. The Journal of Thoracic and Cardiovascular Surgery. 2014;**147**(1):6-14

[9] Rao PN, Kumar AS. Aortic valve replacement through right thoracotomy. Texas Heart Institute Journal. 1993; **20**(4):307-308

[10] Van Praet KM, van Kampen A, Kofler M, et al. Minimally invasive surgical aortic valve replacement: The RALT approach. Journal of Cardiac Surgery. 2020;**35**(9):2341-2346

[11] Nguyen TC, Terwelp MD, Thourani VH, et al. Clinical trends in surgical, minimally invasive and transcatheter aortic valve replacement. European Journal of Cardio-Thoracic Surgery. 2017;**51**(6):1086-1092

[12] Ramlawi B, Bedeir K, Lamelas J. Aortic valve surgery: Minimally invasive options. Methodist DeBakey Cardiovascular Journal. 2016;**12**(1): 27-32

[13] Glauber M, Miceli A, Gilmanov D, et al. Right anterior minithoracotomy versus conventional aortic valve replacement: A propensity score matched study. The Journal of Thoracic and Cardiovascular Surgery. 2013; **145**(5):1222-1226

[14] Bowdish ME, Hui DS, Cleveland JD, et al. A comparison of aortic valve replacement via an anterior right minithoracotomy with standard sternotomy: A propensity score analysis of 492 patients. European Journal of Cardio-Thoracic Surgery. 2016;**49**(2): 456-463

[15] Stolinski J, Plicner D, Grudzien G, et al. A comparison of minimally invasive and standard aortic valve replacement. The Journal of Thoracic and Cardiovascular Surgery. 2016; **152**(4):1030-1039

[16] Gilmanov D, Solinas D, Farneti PA, et al. Minimally invasive aortic valve replacement: 12-year single center experience. Annals of Cardiothoracic Surgery. 2015;**4**(2):160-169

[17] Ghanta RK, Lapar DJ, Kern JA, et al. Minimally invasive aortic valve

replacement provides equivalent outcomes at reduced cost compared with conventional aortic valve replacement: A real-world multi-institutional analysis. The Journal of Thoracic and Cardiovascular Surgery. 2015;**149**(4):1060-1065

[18] Semsroth S, Matteucci Gothe R, Rodriguez Raith Y, et al. Comparison of two minimally invasive techniques and median sternotomy in aortic valve replacement. The Annals of Thoracic Surgery. 2017;**104**(3):877-883

[19] Fattouch K, Moscarelli M, Del Giglio M, et al. Non-sutureless minimally invasive aortic valve replacement: Mini-sternotomy versus mini-thoracotomy: A series of 1130 patients. Interactive Cardiovascular and Thoracic Surgery. 2016;**23**(2):253-258

[20] Wu Y, Jiang W, Li D, et al. Surgery of ascending aorta with complex procedures for aortic dissection through upper mini-sternotomy versus conventional sternotomy. Journal of Cardiothoracic Surgery. 2020;**15**(1):57

[21] Lamelas J, Chen PC, Loor G, et al. Successful use of sternal-sparing minimally invasive surgery for proximal ascending aortic pathology. The Annals of Thoracic Surgery. 2018;**106**(3):742-748

[22] Rayner TA, Harrison S, Rival P, et al. Minimally invasive versus conventional surgery of the ascending aorta and root: A systematic review and meta-analysis. European Journal of Cardio-Thoracic Surgery. 2020;**57**(1):8-17

[23] Staromlynski J, Kowalewski M, Sarnowski W, et al. Midterm results of less invasive approach to ascending aorta and aortic root surgery. Journal of Thoracic Disease. 2020;**12**(11):6446-6457

[24] Shuhaiber J. Technology for new surgical aortic valve replacement: Current evidence and future directions. Journal of Thoracic Disease. 2018;**10**(12):6392-6395

Section 3

Pulmonary Valve

Chapter 3

Surgical Options for Pulmonary Valve Pathology in the Current Era

Sameh M. Said

Abstract

Pulmonary valve pathology occurs mostly in the settings of congenital heart disease whether primary or as the result of repair of a variety of congenital heart defects. Acquired pulmonary valve disorders, albeit rare, can occur in the settings of endocarditis, tumors, carcinoid syndrome, or rheumatic fever. Surgical options include repair and replacement of pulmonary valve. Several options for replacement are available, which can be tailored based on the patient's clinical profile and the primary valve pathology. In this chapter, we present the surgical options that are currently available for pulmonary valve disorders and the current outcomes.

Keywords: pulmonary valve replacement, endocarditis, carcinoid syndrome, congenital pulmonary valve stenosis, pulmonary regurgitation, bioprosthesis, mechanical prosthesis, Ozaki

1. Introduction

A variety of congenital and acquired pathologies results in pulmonary valve (PV) disease that necessitates intervention. The types of this intervention depend on the main pathology with transcatheter options such as balloon valvuloplasty and transcatheter pulmonary valve implantation gaining popularity in the current era, especially in the congenital settings to delay the need for a sternotomy or repeat surgery. Surgical options include open valvotomy for congenital pulmonary valve stenosis and pulmonary valve repair or replacement for many other pathologies. Several replacement options are available currently such as homografts, bioprostheses, and mechanical prostheses with long-term data. Other novel techniques such as intra-operative reconstruction of pulmonary valve leaflets using autologous or bovine pericardium and creation of hand-made valved conduits are being used but no long-term data are available for these techniques.

The focus of this chapter will be on discussing the several surgical options that are currently used to repair or replace the pulmonary valve and the different surgical approaches that are being used with reviewing the literature regarding outcomes. Discussion of the various pathologies involving the pulmonary valve, or the right ventricular outflow tract, is beyond the scope of this chapter.

IntechOpen

2. Etiology of pulmonary valve disease

- Congenital
  - Primary
    - Pulmonary stenosis
    - Pulmonary atresia
  - Secondary to surgical treatment of congenital lesions
    - Pulmonary regurgitation after tetralogy of Fallot repair
    - Homograft dysfunctions:
      - Following Ross procedure
      - Homografts used for reconstruction of the right ventricular outflow tract (RVOT):
        - Pulmonary atresia
        - Complex forms of tetralogy of Fallot
        - Truncus arteriosus
- Acquired
  - Carcinoid heart disease
  - Endocarditis
  - Pulmonary artery aneurysms
  - Tumors
  - Rheumatic heart disease

3. Surgical options for pulmonary valve pathology

3.1 Open (surgical) pulmonary valvotomy

Although transcatheter pulmonary balloon valvuloplasty is becoming a gold standard for isolated congenital pulmonary valve stenosis, surgical (open) pulmonary valvotomy may be required in some cases that are most commonly associated with pulmonary annular hypoplasia (**Figure 1**). The advantage of the open technique is the ability to relief the right ventricular outflow tract (RVOT) obstruction in a controlled fashion *via* splitting the commissures of the pulmonary valve without causing significant regurgitation. It is also useful in addressing associated pulmonary annular hypoplasia *via* the use of a concomitant transannular patch with

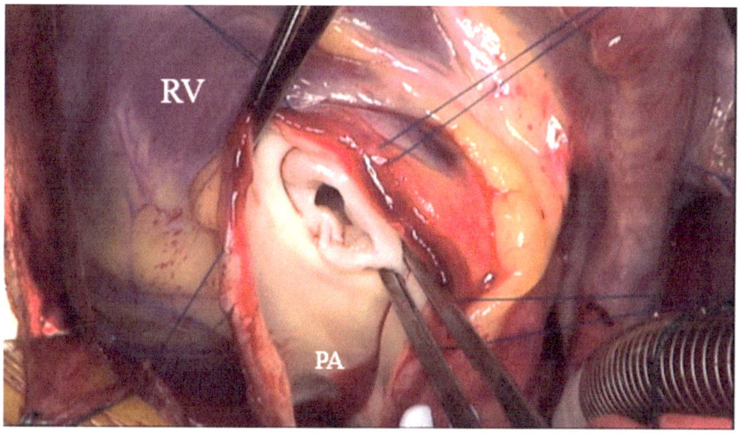

Figure 1.
Intraoperative photo in an infant with isolated congenital pulmonary valve stenosis and hypoplastic pulmonary annulus. Notice the classic bicuspid pulmonary valve with fused commissures. RV: right ventricle; PA: pulmonary artery.

or without reconstruction of a monocusp leaflet. This technique is reported to have long-term excellent results in selected patients [1].

3.2 Pulmonary valve repair

Pulmonary valve repair is possible in selected congenital or acquired cases of pulmonary regurgitation. In the patients who underwent repair of tetralogy of Fallot (TOF) *via* a transannular patch with preservation of the native pulmonary leaflets and present later with dilated pulmonary artery and free pulmonary regurgitation, it is possible to remove the part of the transannular patch and bring the remaining leaflets together anteriorly thus reconstructing the anterior commissure and creating a bicuspid pulmonary valve [2]. In a previous report of 13 patients who underwent TOF repair using a transannular patch and present for pulmonary valve replacement (PVR), it was possible to avoid a prosthesis by repairing the pulmonary valve according to the technique described above [2]. The degree of regurgitation was markedly decreased in all patients and continued during the follow-up period. It is also possible to create a new leaflet from the autologous or bovine pericardium to form a tricuspid pulmonary valve if the other remaining two leaflets are of good quality thus avoiding the use of a prosthesis/homograft.

3.3 Pulmonary valve replacement

Although most valve procedures performed annually involve the aortic and/or mitral valves, the need for pulmonary valve replacement (PVR) is increasing due to the increase in patients with congenital heart disease who survive to adulthood. Because of the improved postoperative care and long-term survival of children undergoing repair of congenital heart defects, it is reasonable to predict that the problem of young adults who have developed sequelae of pulmonary regurgitation after repair of tetralogy of Fallot or neonatal/infant interventions for pulmonary stenosis or atresia will be seen with increasing frequency. In general, most authors recommend the use of bioprostheses or homografts for PVR in children and young adults [3].

A wide variety of materials have been utilized for PVR and or reconstruction of the RVOT. The most commonly used materials include autologous or bovine pericardium, bioprosthetic (bovine or porcine) or mechanical valves, Dacron conduits/grafts, bovine jugular veins, and homograft (aortic and pulmonary).

3.3.1 Autologous pericardial reconstruction (Ozaki)

The autologous pericardium has been used for decades to create aortic and/or pulmonary valve leaflets (one or more) and more recently has been used to create three-leaflet aortic valves *via* standardized templates (Ozaki procedure) [4]. This procedure began in the adult population but has recently widely spread to the pediatric patients with aortic valve pathology with good initial and mid-term results in some series [5].

More recently, the same procedure has been used to create three-leaflet pulmonary valves for PVR (**Figures 2A–F** and **3**). Limited literatures are available for the Ozaki outcome in the pulmonary position and the majority of these are case reports using autologous pericardium [6] or bovine pericardium [7]. This was used in the setting of pulmonary artery aneurysm [8], endocarditis, and free pulmonary regurgitation after previous pulmonary valvotomy. We have utilized the Ozaki templates to create three leaflet pulmonary valves for an infant who was born with congenital pulmonary stenosis and hypoplastic annulus and in another child who underwent late repair of tetralogy of Fallot with pulmonary stenosis.

3.3.2 Valved conduits

Valved conduits used during the repair of a variety of congenital heart defects, most commonly tetralogy of Fallot with pulmonary atresia, truncus arteriosus, and Rastelli procedure for (corrected) transposition of the great arteries with pulmonary outflow tract obstruction. These conduits include homografts (aortic/pulmonary/femoral vein), xenografts (bovine jugular vein), and synthetic (Dacron

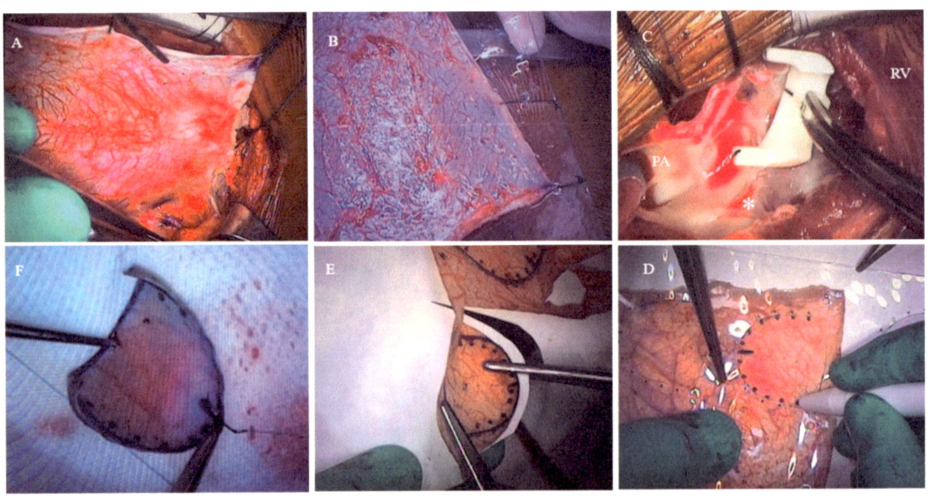

Figure 2.
Intraoperative photos demonstrating the Ozaki technique for reconstruction of a new pulmonary valve using the autologous pericardium. (A) A large sheet of the anterior pericardium is harvested once the sternotomy is performed, (B) the pericardium is then mounted on the plate provided with the Ozaki set and is treated with glutaraldehyde 0.6% for 3 minutes, (C) the main pulmonary artery and the right ventricular outflow tract are opened longitudinally and remnants of the pulmonary valve leaflets are resected and the Ozaki sizers are used to determine the size of the future pericardial leaflets and to mark the suture lines and determine the location of the commissures, (D) the pericardial leaflets are marked using the Ozaki template, (E) the leaflets are cut with scissors, and (F) suturing is begun with running polypropylene along the marked lines in the right ventricular outflow tract. RV: right ventricle.

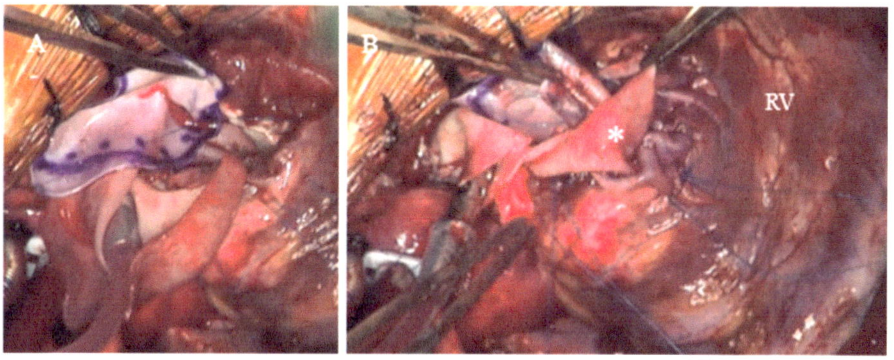

Figure 3.
Intraoperative photos showing the rest of the steps for the Ozaki reconstruction of the pulmonary valve. (A) Pericardial leaflets are sewn in with running polypropylene sutures, and (B) two leaflets along the posterior native annulus and the anterior leaflet is sewn to the undersurface of the pericardial patch (asterisk) that is used to augment the right ventricular outflow tract and the main pulmonary artery. RV: right ventricle.

conduit, expanded polytetrafluoroethylene [e-PTFE]). Several factors affect the choice of any of these valved conduits such as the age of the patient, the original pathology, previous procedure/conduit used, and availability.

3.3.3 Homografts

Homografts continued to remain the most commonly used conduits for RVOT reconstruction. A variety of these homografts have been used including aortic, pulmonary (**Figure 4**), and more recently valved femoral veins. The advantages include its availability in smaller sizes and the lack of the rigidity associated with other prostheses, which make them suitable conduits for neonates, infants, and small children. Downsides include long-term calcifications, cost, and limited availability in many countries. We reserve the use of homografts for infants and small

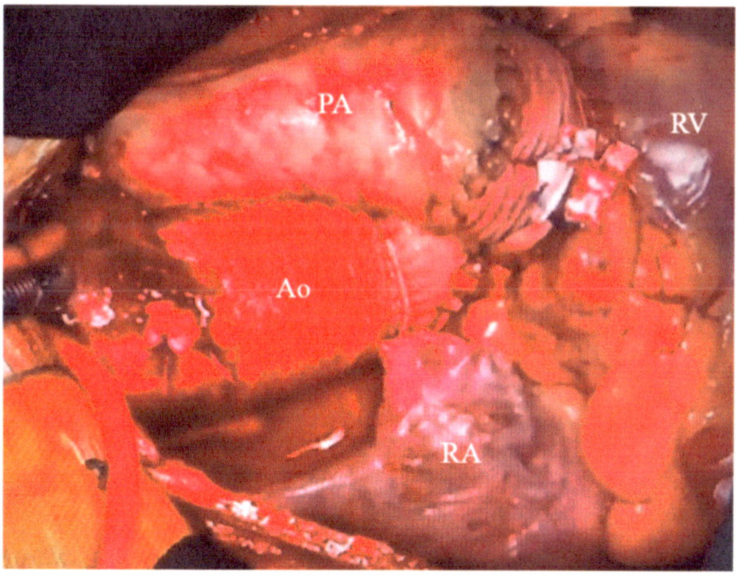

Figure 4.
Intraoperative photo for a patient who underwent a Ross procedure with a pulmonary homograft used to establish the right ventricular-to-pulmonary arterial confluence continuity. RV: right ventricle, Ao: ascending aorta, PA: pulmonary artery homograft, RA: right atrium.

children due to the absence of suitable size prostheses in this age and for those with endocarditis as well.

3.3.4 Expanded polytetrafluoroethylene (e-PTFE) (Gore-Tex) conduits

Handmade expanded e-PTFE valves have been used with good results for RVOT reconstruction. The main advantages of these handmade conduits are related to their availability and lack of calcifications or immunological reactions, which may have the potential to prolong the longevity of these conduits. Current data do not show the inferiority of these conduits to homografts or bovine jugular veins. In fact, they have good biocompatibility and there was no evidence of calcifications in excised e-PTFE valves [9]. We personally do not have experience with this technique.

3.3.5 Biological prostheses

The vast majority of children and young adults who require PVR receive a biological valve. These prostheses carry the advantage of good durability in the pulmonary position and avoidance of long-term anticoagulation.

3.3.6 Mechanical prostheses

While bioprostheses are the most commonly used prostheses for PVR, the need for repeat operation is inevitable in children and young adults with congenital heart disease and mechanical prostheses may be considered in selected clinical scenarios to minimize the risks involved with repeat operations. The operative risk of mortality increases from 2% at the first repeat sternotomy compared with 4.7% at a fourth sternotomy [10]. Furthermore, Morishita and colleagues demonstrated a fourth time sternotomy to be a predictor of resternotomy-related injury (hazard ratio, 4.31) [11].

Most of those who are considered for mechanical PVR had a congenital diagnosis and underwent multiple previous sternotomies in the past (**Figure** 5).

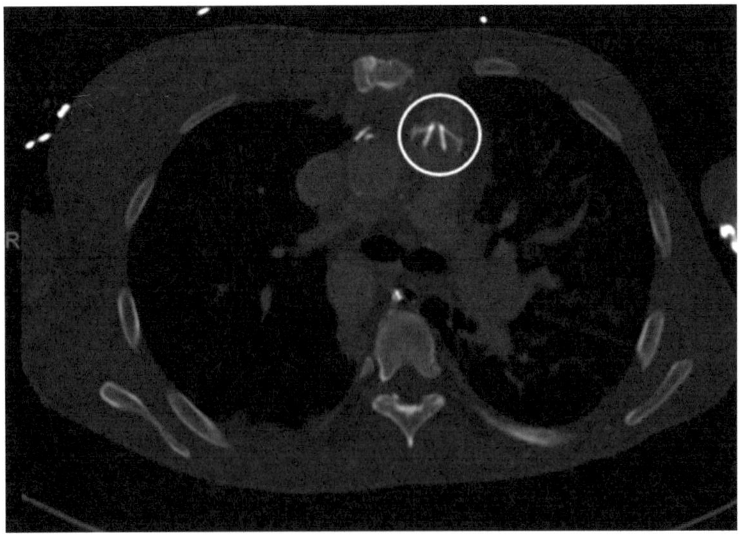

Figure 5.
Computed tomography scan in a patient who underwent multiple previous sternotomies for an initial Rastelli procedure with subsequent multiple pulmonary conduits changes and has a bileaflet mechanical prosthesis in the pulmonary position (white circle).

Although mechanical prostheses are durable, the need for higher-level anticoagulation carries its own risks, but recent reports suggest that with proper anticoagulation and careful monitoring, the risk of prosthetic thrombosis or dysfunction is low.

The issue of the performance of a mechanical prosthesis in the pulmonary position remains a matter of debate as there are no precise criteria for the selection of patients in whom this prosthesis would be well suited. We believe the ideal patient for mechanical PVR is the patient who underwent multiple previous sternotomies and/or requires anticoagulation for another reason such as a left-sided mechanical prosthesis. This patient population includes those with repaired truncus arteriosus, prior Ross procedure, and occasionally repaired tetralogy of Fallot. Other indications may include those who demonstrated poor durability of bioprostheses.

In every case where a mechanical prosthesis is considered, the ultimate treatment decision is individualized after weighing the risks of reoperation if a bioprosthesis is chosen, with the potential bleeding/thrombotic risks if a mechanical prosthesis is chosen.

4. Preoperative evaluation

Associated defects that commonly need to be addressed at the time of PVR include tricuspid valve repair, patch pulmonary arterioplasties, closure of residual shunts, and arrhythmia surgery.

Preoperative transthoracic echocardiography (TTE), computed tomography (CT) scan, or magnetic resonance imaging (MRI) are routinely performed. Cross-sectional imaging is helpful to determine the relationship of mediastinal structures especially the aorta and/or extracardiac conduits to the sternum and in assessing the pulmonary arterial anatomy. Coronary artery evaluation may be needed in certain circumstances to rule out obstructive coronary artery disease or coronary anomalies especially ones that may change the surgical plan regarding the PVR technique. Hemodynamic data from cardiac catheterization may be needed to complement other studies when there is uncertainty about the anatomy or ventricular function.

Intraoperative transesophageal echocardiography (TEE) is routinely performed before and after cardiopulmonary bypass with or without intraoperative direct pressure measurement across the right ventricular outflow tract.

5. Surgical approaches

5.1 Median (Re-do) sternotomy

Primary or repeat sternotomy has been the most commonly used approach. Technical aspects of repeat sternotomy with or without peripheral cannulation have been discussed previously [12].

5.2 Left posterolateral thoracotomy

Left posterolateral thoracotomy has been used as an alternate to sternotomy/ repeat sternotomy for PVR [13]. With the patient in the modified right lateral decubitus position, the chest is usually entered through the left fourth/fifth intercostal space. Normothermic cardiopulmonary bypass is established *via* the femoral vessels. It is important to rule out the presence of any intracardiac shunts before proceeding with this approach. The right ventricular outflow tract and main pulmonary artery are identified, and once the pulmonary artery is incised, the PVR is proceeded as described below.

5.3 Minimally invasive left anterior thoracotomy incision

We have utilized left anterior minithoracotomy as an alternative approach to sternotomy for PVR in selected patients who required isolated PVR and in the absence of intracardiac shunts. This approach carries the advantage of being less invasive with rapid recovery, but careful patient selection is required. It is not advisable in the presence of previous pulmonary conduits, but it can be useful in cases where hostile mediastinum is encountered after multiple previous surgeries or in the presence of a large aorta in close proximity to the sternum, which increases the risk of repeat sternotomy.

We have previously published our technique that can be used in both primary and reoperative settings [14] (**Figures 6A–F** and **7A** and **B**). In summary, the patient is positioned supine, prepped, and draped as for standard median sternotomy. A 6-cm horizontal incision is performed through the left third or fourth intercostal space. In primary operative settings, the left lung is gently retracted to expose the pericardium, which is then incised anterior to the left phrenic nerve to expose the RVOT and the main pulmonary artery. In re-operative settings, the left lung is usually adherent to the RVOT and/or the previously placed transannular patch if the pericardium was not closed after the first procedure and will need to be dissected off the main pulmonary artery and RVOT.

Cardiopulmonary bypass is established *via* the femoral vessels (open/percutaneously cannulated) at normothermia. It is important to achieve adequate right

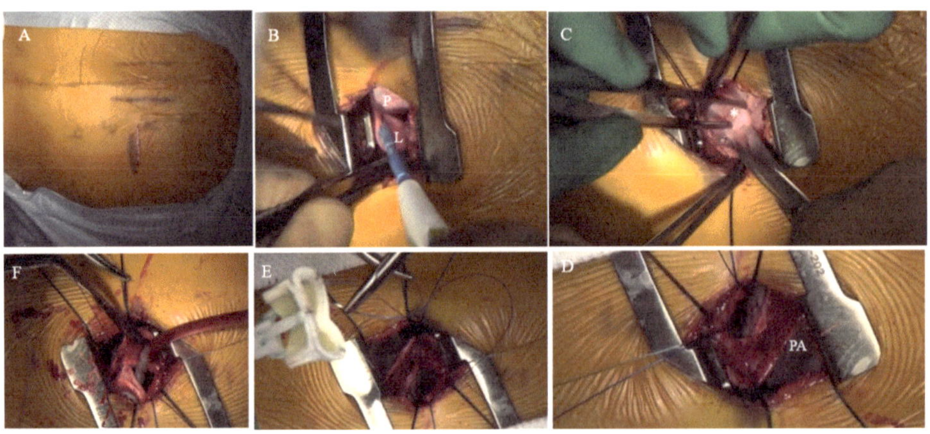

Figure 6.
Intraoperative photos demonstrating the technical steps for pulmonary valve replacement via a minimally invasive left anterior thoracotomy. (A) The patient is positioned supine and a 6-cm horizontal skin incision is created along the left parasternal border along the left third/fourth ribs, (B) the left chest is entered through the left third/fourth intercostal space, and the left lung is retracted medially to expose the pericardium or the previously placed transannular patch, (C) in reoperative settings, pleural adhesions (asterisk) need to be taken down to free the lung from the right ventricular outflow tract, (D) cardiopulmonary bypass is established via the femoral vessels and once the heart is decompressed, the main pulmonary artery/transannular patch is incised longitudinally to expose the pulmonary valve, (E) remnants of the pulmonary valve leaflets are excised, annulus is sized and a new bioprosthesis is seated along the posterior annulus using running polypropylene suture, and (F) the majority of the prosthesis is seated along the native pulmonary annulus, while the anterior portion will be secured to the pericardial patch that will be used to augment the right ventricular outflow tract. P: pericardium, L: left lung, PA: main pulmonary artery.

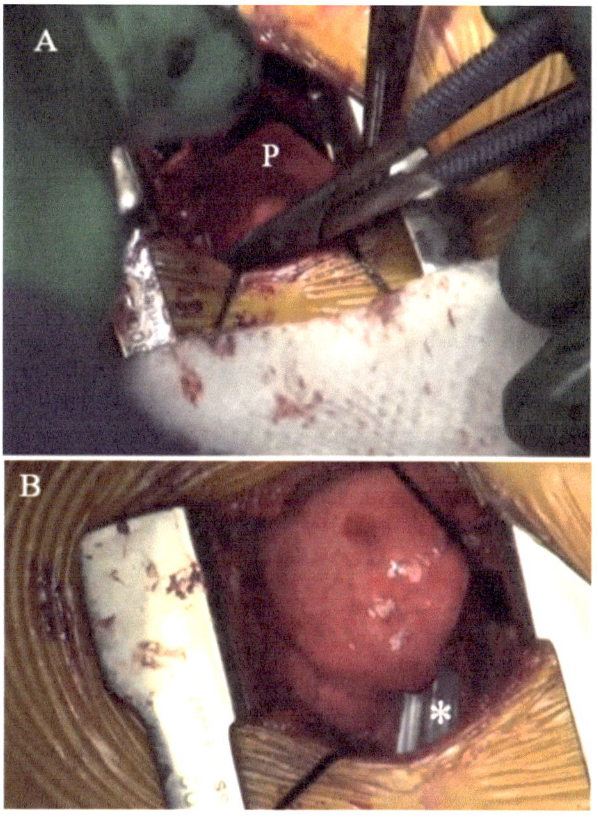

Figure 7.
Intraoperative photos showing the remaining steps in pulmonary valve replacement via a left anterior thoracotomy. (A) A pericardial patch is commonly used to complete the augmentation of the main pulmonary artery and right ventricular outflow tract and the prosthesis is sewn to the undersurface of this patch with a running polypropylene suture, and (B) once the reconstruction is completed, the patient is weaned off cardiopulmonary bypass, and a single chest tube (asterisk) is placed, and the incision is closed in layers in the standard fashion. P: pericardial patch.

heart decompression during this procedure owing to the limited exposure. Along with routine use of vacuum-assisted venous drainage, we prefer to use a multistage venous cannula that is inserted *via* the common femoral vein and advanced all the way up to the superior vena cava. A vertical incision is made along the previous transannular patch/main pulmonary artery and remnants of pulmonary valve leaflets are excised if present. The PVR is then continued as described below. The right side of the heart is then deaired, and the patient is weaned off cardiopulmonary bypass. Once TEE is satisfactory, the groin is decannulated and femoral vessels are repaired. A single chest drain is placed and both groin and chest incisions are then closed in layers. The patient is typically extubated in the operating room at the end of the procedure.

Our experience with this technique is in its early phase, but we have performed the procedure in 6 patients (the youngest at age 13 years; 4 with previous tetralogy of Fallot repair). The procedure was feasible, with no conversion to open sternotomy in any. There was no early or late mortality. One patient developed a femoral artery pseudoaneurysm during follow-up due to percutaneous cannulation and required late repair. The length of stay averaged 2 days [15]. We believe that weight more than 30 kg is necessary for satisfactory groin vessel cannulation.

6. Surgical techniques of pulmonary valve replacement

6.1 Sternal re-entry

Basics of primary or repeat sternotomy are followed. Sternal re-entry can be challenging, especially in the presence of a right-sided pathology (e.g., pulmonary hypertension, enlarged right heart structures, or extracardiac conduit). We prefer the oscillating saw for repeat sternotomy, although a craniotome can also be used.

The decision to expose the femoral vessels versus cannulating them and initiating cardiopulmonary bypass to facilitate sternotomy is individualized and is dependent on the experience of the surgeon. Groin cannulation can be performed *via* a cut down with or without percutaneous right internal jugular to superior vena cava cannulation, which allows establishing complete cardiopulmonary bypass. Special attention is made to ensure adequate antegrade perfusion and adequate venous return of the lower extremity. This may require a chimney graft on the femoral artery. Axillary artery cannulation is also an option and is preferred if concomitant aortic surgery is being performed. If it is necessary to initiate cardiopulmonary bypass before or during sternal reentry, it is important to maintain a positive central venous pressure to avoid potential air embolism, which can occur if there is inadvertent entry into the right heart in the presence of an intracardiac shunt.

The procedure can be performed with aortic and a single-venous cannulation at normothermia in the absence of concomitant cardiac pathology that needs concomitant repair. It is commonly performed on the beating heart without cardioplegic arrest in the absence of intracardiac shunts. However, a short period of aortic cross-clamping and cardioplegia may be needed in challenging cases where heavily calcified or scarred RVOT patches or conduits are present to allow safe decalcification and adequate debridement before removing the cross-clamp and completing the PVR or the new conduit placement on a beating heart.

6.2 Pulmonary valve reconstruction with autologous pericardium (pulmonary Ozaki)

The basic principle of the technique in harvesting the autologous pericardium and creating the leaflets and sewing them is similar to the Ozaki technique described for aortic valve replacement.

However, there are important anatomical differences between the aortic and pulmonary roots that required modification of the technique to facilitate exposure and leaflet placement. Three possible ways to apply this technique for pulmonary valve reconstruction are as follows:

- If the pulmonary artery and root are adequate, the main pulmonary artery can be completely transected, and the leaflets are sized with the appropriate Ozaki sizers and suture lines are marked at the native pulmonary annulus in a similar fashion to the aortic procedure. The leaflets are then sewn in a similar fashion to the aortic technique; then, the pulmonary artery continuity is re-established.

- A second strategy is to build a valved conduit with pericardial leaflets sewn inside a Dacron graft on the back table; then, the conduit is implanted in a similar fashion to a standard pulmonary conduit.

- More commonly, the patient is presented with a hypoplastic pulmonary annulus that needs to be enlarged. A longitudinal pulmonary arteriotomy is performed, and the two posterior leaflets are created along the pulmonary annulus/RVOT. The RVOT is enlarged with a pericardial patch in a way similar to the transannular patch technique. This patch is extended up to the future sinotubular junction, and the third leaflet is then sewn to the pericardial patch and the commissures are created followed by completing the augmentation of the main pulmonary artery with the remainder of the patch.

6.3 Biological/mechanical prosthesis

6.3.1 Isolated PVR

6.3.1.1 Previous transannular patch

The most common scenario occurs with a dilated right ventricular outflow tract from the previous repair of tetralogy of Fallot with a transannular patch (**Figure 8A–D**). In the setting, the patch is opened longitudinally and stay sutures are placed on both sides. Most commonly, the incision is extended proximally into the RVOT and distally into the proximal left main branch pulmonary artery. Pathological/remnant pulmonary valve cusps are resected if present. An appropriately sized bovine pericardial patch (our preference) is then chosen and sewn distally to the proximal left main branch pulmonary artery. It is not uncommon that concomitant branch pulmonary arterioplasty is needed in these cases. The patch is sewn in with running polypropylene sutures till the proposed level of the new pulmonary prosthesis is reached.

An appropriately sized prosthesis (biological/mechanical) is chosen and is secured along the native pulmonary annulus posteriorly with running polypropylene suture (interrupted sutures with or without pledgets may be used sometimes based on the tissue quality). It is critical to avoid deep sutures along the pulmonary annulus due to the close proximity of the left main coronary artery.

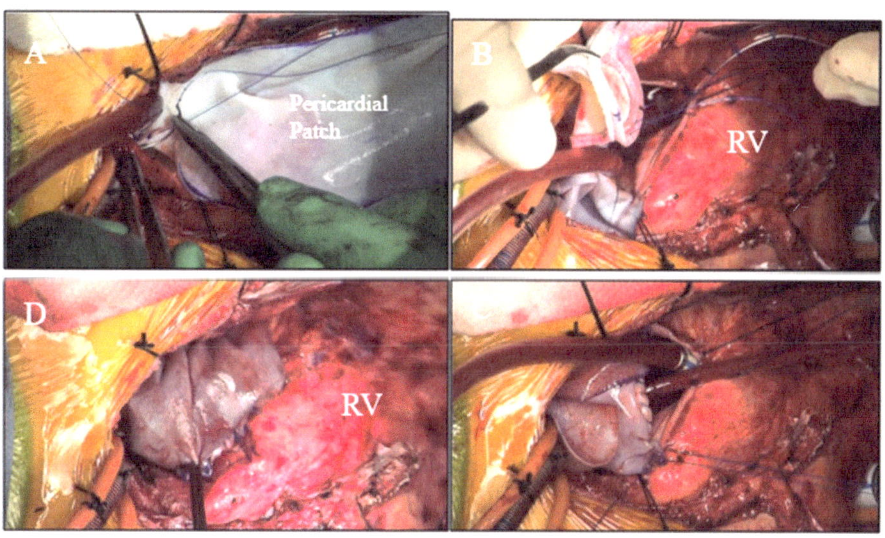

Figure 8.
Intraoperative photos showing the most commonly used technique for pulmonary valve replacement. (A) A longitudinal incision is created along the main pulmonary artery and is extended proximally into the right ventricular outflow tract and distally usually to the proximal left main pulmonary artery. A large pericardial patch is then sued to augment the main pulmonary artery is extended down to the level of the future prosthesis, (B) the prosthesis is secured with a running polypropylene suture along the posterior annulus, (C) the anterior portion of the sewing ring is then secured to the undersurface of the pericardial patch, (D) the remainder of the patch is trimmed and used to complete the right ventricular outflow tract reconstruction. RV: right ventricle.

In fact, in some situations, it is better to place the prosthesis more distally (between the native pulmonary annulus and the pulmonary artery bifurcation) to avoid compromising the left coronary artery. The anterior portion of the sewing ring of the prosthesis is then secured to the undersurface of the patch with a running suture. It is important to carefully think about the orientation of the prosthesis before securing it to the undersurface of the patch and especially when it is a biological one due to its larger profile that can create a higher gradient across its path if not oriented properly. The prosthesis should be tilted posteriorly toward the pulmonary bifurcation. Also, it is important to have some redundancy in the pericardial patch proximal and distal to the prosthesis to ensure no gradient is created due to a tight patch. This completes the prosthesis securement in the outflow tract. The rest of the bovine pericardial patch is then trimmed and sewn to the RVOT to complete its reconstruction.

6.3.1.2 Dilated pulmonary root with no patch

If the main pulmonary artery/outflow tract is dilated or in the presence of a pulmonary artery aneurysm, our technique is different. A transverse pulmonary arteriotomy is created, and a running or interrupted suture technique is used to secure the prosthesis similar to a standard aortic valve replacement. The pulmonary arteriotomy is then closed with a running polypropylene suture.

6.4 Valved pulmonary conduit

This is commonly used to replace a failed or dysfunctional conduit that was placed in a previous operation as a part of the initial repair of congenital heart defects such as tetralogy of Fallot with pulmonary atresia, truncus arteriosus, and post-Ross and Rastelli procedures.

It is critical to keep in mind the location of the left main coronary artery (posterior) and the left anterior descending coronary artery (lateral) in relation to the conduit especially when anatomical details are unclear in the setting of repeat

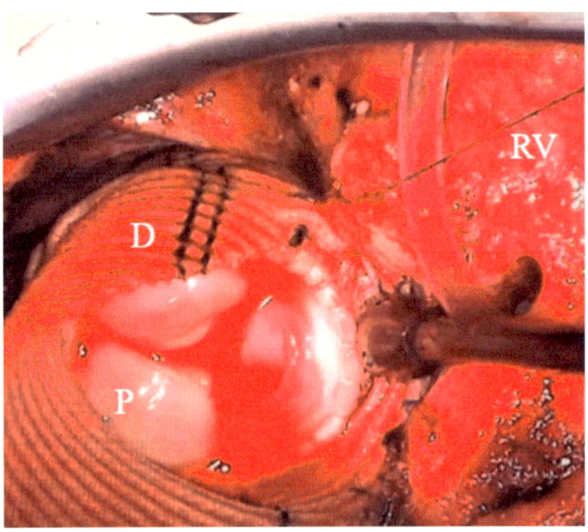

Figure 9.
Intraoperative photo showing a surgically created pulmonary conduit by placing a bioprosthesis inside a Dacron tube graft which is sewn proximally and distally to the right ventricular outflow tract and the pulmonary arterial confluence respectively. RV: right ventricle, D: Dacron tube graft, P: pulmonary bioprosthesis.

operations. The conduit itself while in most cases is located to the left of the sternum, and in certain congenital heart defects, it may be immediately behind the sternum, or in the midline such as cases of the previous repair of truncus arteriosus. This may require modification of the surgical technique during reoperation or initiation of cardiopulmonary bypass *via* peripheral cannulation to avoid injury to the conduit during repeat sternotomy. The majority of these conduits (homografts) are calcified to various degrees, which may increase the difficulty during the replacement. It may also require a complete explantation of the conduit to be able to replace a new one.

We have used different techniques in these situations depending on the quality of the previous conduit and the degree of calcification present:

- A longitudinal incision is placed in the anterior aspect of the conduit, while its posterior wall is kept intact, which minimizes injury to the left main coronary artery. After adequate debridement and decalcification, the new prosthesis is placed with a roof of pericardial patch similar to the technique described in the case of the transannular patch.

- If the previous conduit was a Dacron conduit, it can be dissected from the external fibrous peel and excised. It is important to minimize dissection of the floor and preserve the thick fibrous peel to allow sturdy suture placement.

- The position of the new prosthesis is critically important. In general, we place the prosthesis distally toward the pulmonary confluence, which minimizes potential compression of the left main coronary artery. Alternatively, the prosthesis can be placed more proximally near the level of the native pulmonary annulus.

- In some scenarios, the old conduit can be completely excised, and, in these cases, there is a lack of continuity between the RVOT and the pulmonary confluence. We then create a new valved conduit using a biological/mechanical prosthesis inside a Dacron tube graft (**Figure 9**), which is then sewn proximally and distally to the RVOT and the pulmonary arterial confluence respectably.

Regarding mechanical prostheses, it is important not to oversize them even if there is enough room to place a large prosthesis. Having a mild gradient across the prosthesis (10-15 mmHg) and a higher velocity facilitate leaflet mobility in a more effective way. When the prosthesis is oversized and the gradient is quite low (<5 mmHg), then only one disk may open properly, while the other is poorly moving, which increases the risk of thrombosis.

Finally, the heart is adequately de-aired and cardiopulmonary bypass is discontinued. Post-procedure TEE is performed, and direct pressure measurements of the right ventricular and pulmonary arterial pressures are obtained.

7. Outcomes

7.1 Valved conduits

Dacron conduits create thick intimal peel that requires explantation at the time of repeat operations. Homografts and bovine jugular veins show variable degrees of durability, but early degeneration and calcifications are sometimes inevitable (**Figure 10**). Added to this is their limited availability in many countries.

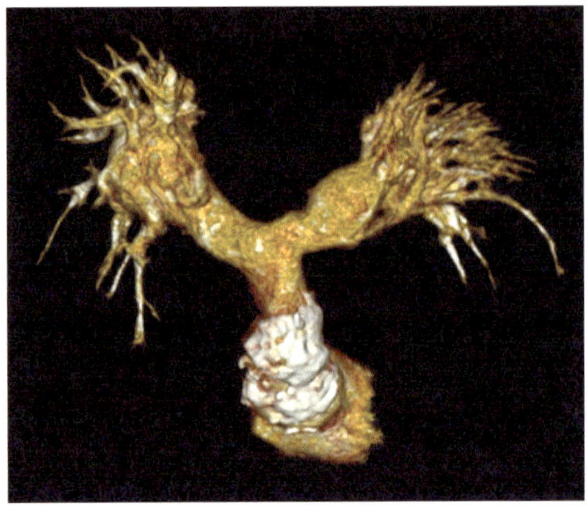

Figure 10.
Preoperative CT scan showing calcified bovine jugular vein graft in patient who underwent repeat sternotomy for pulmonary conduit replacement.

A multicenter study in Japan included 794 patients (aged 14 days to 56.8 years old) in which e-PTFE valves were used for RVOT reconstruction at 52 Japanese institutes had a mean follow-up of 3.6 years (maximum 10 years) [16]. The e-PTFE was in the form of fan-shaped valved conduits and patches with bulging sinuses. The freedom from reoperation at 10 years was 95.4% in patients with conduits and 92.3% in those with patches. No or mild pulmonary regurgitation was present in 95 and 79.6% of those with conduits and those with patches, respectively.

7.2 Biological prostheses

In general, there are conflicting reports in the literature regarding the durability of various prostheses in the pulmonary position. Bando et al. observed that 94% of homografts have good function after 5 years; however, almost 25% had evidence of moderate-to-severe calcifications (**Figure 11A** and **B**) [17].

Regarding bioprosthetic conduits, a failure rate of 15% of 3 years was observed in the study by Cleveland et al. and calculated that 55% would have avoided a reoperation at 5 years [18].

In the study by Batlivala et al., the authors compared bioprostheses and homograft conduits in the pulmonary position [19]. This included 254 patients aged 10–21 years old. The median follow-up was 4.4 years. Freedom from valvar dysfunction was 72% ± 4% at 5 years and 48% ± 8% at 10 years. Freedom from RVOT re-interventions was 90% ± 3%, and 67% ± 5% at 5 and 10 years, respectively. No differences were present between bioprosthesis and homografts.

7.3 Mechanical prostheses

In a study from Mayo Clinic, 59 patients underwent mechanical PVR between 1965 and 2013, and no valve thrombosis was observed in the settings of adequate anticoagulation with Warfarin. The maximum follow-up in this study extended to 20 years with no reoperations related to pannus formation, paravalvular leak, endocarditis, valve thrombosis, or prosthetic dysfunction.

The range of reported thrombosis for a mechanical PVR varies from 25 to 80% [20]. These thrombotic complications were reported with bileaflet mechanical prostheses, and none was reported in those with a tilting-disk prosthesis, although literature on this topic is spared in general. The reported complication rate of a bileaflet

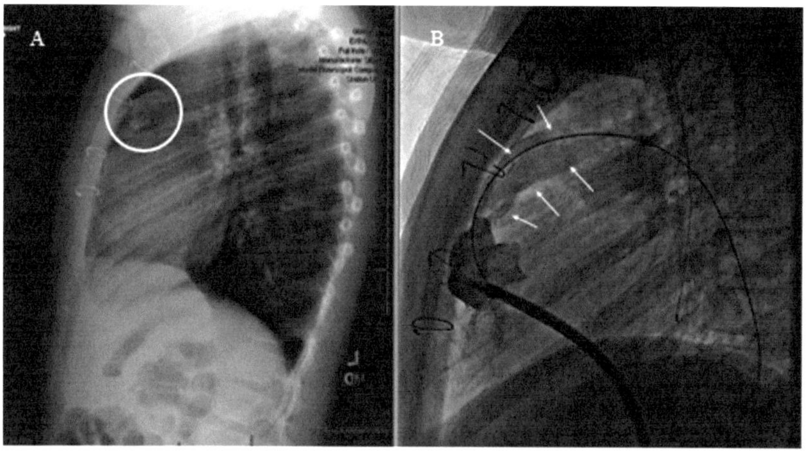

Figure 11.
Preoperative images of a patient who had previous aortic homograft placed in the right ventricular outflow tract for repair of tetralogy of Fallot with pulmonary atresia. (A) Chest X ray showing extensive and complete calcifications of the homograft pulmonary conduit (white circle), (B) which is confirmed by preoperative cardiac catheterization (multiple white arrows). Notice the close proximity of the pulmonary conduit to the back of the sternum.

prosthesis in the pulmonary position has been about 35%. The majority of these thrombotic events were observed in those who were not adequately anticoagulated with Warfarin. Taken together, the frequency of thrombosis if the patient was not maintained on Warfarin was 41% (15 of 37 prostheses failed); however, if the patient is adequately anticoagulated, the rate of thrombosis dropped to 3.5% [21, 22]. These observations are seen also in the series reported by Freling et al., which spanned 26 years and included 66 patients [23]. Actuarial freedom from reoperation was 96% at 5 years and 89% at 10 years.

A meta-analysis of 299 patients from 19 observational studies by Dunne et al. documented nonstructural deterioration and valve thrombosis rates of 1.5 and 2.2%, respectively [24]. Redo surgery was needed in 0.9%, and thrombolysis was used in 0.5%. This is the largest analysis to date and confirms the low incidence of valve dysfunction and thrombosis for mechanical prostheses in the pulmonary position.

8. Conclusions

The pulmonary valve can be affected by a variety of congenital and acquired diseases. Although repair or preservation of the pulmonary valve may be possible in certain cases, replacement is usually required whether in primary or reoperative settings based on the original, pathology affecting the pulmonary valve/RVOT.

Surgical approaches can be through (repeat) sternotomy, left posterolateral thoracotomy, or minimally invasive left anterior minithoracotomy.

Several options are available for the replacement of the pulmonary valve with or without reconstruction of the RVOT. The most commonly used options include homografts and bioprosthetic or mechanical valves. While our first choice as a prosthesis for PVR is a biological valve that facilitates subsequent transcatheter interventions (**Figure 12**), the deciding factor between any of these options depends on the patient's clinical profile especially age, original pathology/indication, prosthesis availability, and future expectations for this patient and therefore, it should be individualized. Other novel strategies such as handmade e-PTFE conduits and autologous pericardial leaflet reconstruction may be considered.

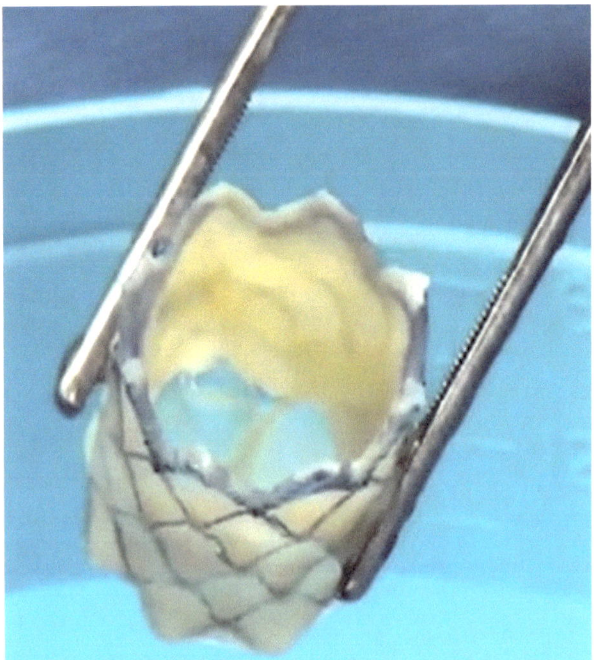

Figure 12.
Melody transcatheter valve is they most commonly used transcatheter option after failed pulmonary bioprostheses and homografts.

Although some of these conduits have long-term data in terms of durability and freedom from reintervention, literatures are limited regarding other techniques and the bottom line is we do not have the ideal pulmonary valve/conduit yet.

Conflict of interest

The author (S.M.S) is a consultant for Cryolife and Stryker.

Author details

Sameh M. Said
Division of Pediatric Cardiovascular Surgery, Masonic Children's Hospital, University of Minnesota, Minneapolis, MN, USA

*Address all correspondence to: ssaid@umn.edu

References

[1] Sekhon S, Barger PM, Abarbanell AM. Outcomes 60 years after surgical valvotomy for isolated congenital pulmonary valve stenosis. Journal of Cardiac Surgery. 2021;**36**:1531-1533

[2] Said SM, Mainwaring RD, Ma M, Tacy T, Hanley FL. Pulmonary valve repair for patients with acquire pulmonary valve insufficiency. The Annals of Thoracic Surgery. 2016;**101**:2294-2301

[3] Rosti L, Murzi B, Colli AM, Festa P, Redaelli S, Havelova L, et al. Mechanical valves in the pulmonary position: A reappraisal. The Journal of Thoracic and Cardiovascular Surgery. 1998;**115**:1074-1079

[4] Ozaki S, Kawase I, Yamashita H, Uchida S, Nozawa Y, Takatoh M, et al. A total of 404 cases of aortic valve reconstruction with glutaraldehyde-treated autologous pericardium. The Journal of Thoracic and Cardiovascular Surgery. 2014;**147**:301-306

[5] Ozaki S, Kawase I, Yamashita H, Uchida S, Takatoh M, Kiyohara N. Midterm outcomes after aortic valve neocuspidization with glutaraldehyde-treated autologous pericardium. The Journal of Thoracic and Cardiovascular Surgery. 2018;**155**:2379-2387

[6] Yepez C, Rios J. Pulmonary valve reconstruction using Ozaki's technique for infective endocarditis. European Journal of Cardio-Thoracic Surgery. 2021;**59**(4):917-919

[7] Baird C, Chavez M, Friedman K. Pulmonary valve reconstruction using the Ozaki leaflet reconstructive techniques. The Annals of Thoracic Surgery. 2021;**111**(1):e19-e21

[8] Takahashi Y, Shibata T, Fujii H, Morisaki A, Sakon Y, Yamane K, et al. Aortic and pulmonary valve reconstruction using autologous pericardium in narrow annuli. The Annals of Thoracic Surgery. 2020;**109**:e13-e15

[9] Ando M, Takahashi Y. Ten-year experience with handmade trileaflet polytetrafluoroethylene valved conduit used for pulmonary reconstruction. The Journal of Thoracic and Cardiovascular Surgery. 2009;**137**:124-131

[10] Brown ML, Dearani JA, Burkhart HM. The adult with congenital heart disease: Medical and surgical considerations for management. Current Opinion in Pediatrics. 2009;**21**:56-61

[11] Morishita K, Kawaharada N, Fukada J, Yamada A, Masaru T, Kuwaki K, et al. Three or more median sternotomies for patients with valve disease: Role of computed tomography. The Annals of Thoracic Surgery. 2003;**75**:1476-1480

[12] Said SM, Dearani JA. Strategies for high-risk reoperations in congenital heart disease. Seminars in Thoracic and Cardiovascular Surgery. Pediatric Cardiac Surgery Annual 2014;**17**(1): 9-21.

[13] Roubertie F, Henaine R, Roques X, Thambo JB. Left posterolateral thoracotomy: An alternative approach for pulmonary valve replacement. The Annals of Thoracic Surgery. 2014;**97**: 691-693

[14] Said SM. Minimally invasive pulmonary valve replacement via left anterior minithoracotomy. JTCVS Techniques. 2020;**6**:127-129

[15] Said SM, Marey G, Hiremath G, Aggarwal V, Kloesel B, Griselli M. Pulmonary valve replacement via left anterior minithoracotomy: Lessons

learned and early experience. Journal of Cardiac Surgery. 2021;**36**(4):1305-1312

[16] Miyazaki T, Yamagishi M, Maeda Y, Yamamoto Y, Taniguchi S, Sasaki Y, et al. Expanded polytetrafluorethylene conduits and patches with bulging sinuses and fan-shaped valve sin right ventricular outflow tract reconstruction: Multicenter study in Japan. The Journal of Thoracic and Cardiovascular Surgery. 2011;**142**:1122-1129

[17] Bando K, Danielson GK, Schaff HV, Mair DD, Julsrud PR, Puga FJ. Outcome of pulmonary and aortic homografts for right ventricular outflow tract reconstruction. The Journal of Thoracic and Cardiovascular Surgery. 1995;**109**:509-518

[18] Cleveland DC, Williams WG, Razzouk AJ, Trusler GA. Failure of cryopreserved valved conduits in the pulmonary circulation. Circulation. 1992;**86**(Suppl):II150-II153

[19] Batlivala S, Emani S, Mayer J, McElhinney DB. Pulmonary valve replacement function in adolescents: A comparison of bioprosthetic valves and homograft conduits. The Annals of Thoracic Surgery. 2012;**93**:2007-2016

[20] Miyamura H, Kanazawa H, Hayashi J, Eguchi S. Thrombosed St. Jude valve prosthesis on the right side of the heart in patients with tetralogy of Fallot. The Journal of Thoracic and Cardiovascular Surgery. 1987;**94**:148-150

[21] Kawachi Y, Masuda M, Tominaga R, Tokunaga K. Comparative study between St. Jude Medical and bioprosthetic valves in the right side of the heart. Japanese Circulation Journal. 1991;**55**:553-562

[22] Haas F, Schreiber C, Horer J, Kostolny M, Holper K, Lange R. Is there a role for mechanical valved conduits in the pulmonary position? The Annals of Thoracic Surgery. 2005;**79**:1662-1668

[23] Freling HG, Ymkje JVS, van Melle JP, Ebels T, Hoendermis E, Berger R, et al. Pulmonary valve replacement: Twenty-six years of experience with mechanical valvar prostheses. The Annals of Thoracic Surgery. 2015;**99**:905-910

[24] Dunne B, Xiao A, Litton E, Andrews D. Mechanical prostheses for right ventricular outflow tract reconstruction: A systematic review and meta-analysis. The Annals of Thoracic Surgery. 2015;**99**:1841-1847

Section 4

Tricuspid Valve

Chapter 4

Tricuspid Valve Repair

Fevzi Sarper Türker, Zeki Temiztürk and Davut Azboy

Abstract

For the previous years, the tricuspid valve (TV), has been studied relatively less than the other heart valves diseases both about pathophysiology, management, surgical intervention, and treatment. However, recent advances in assessment and management of the TV disease have led to redirect the interest in this "forgotten valve." Surgeons often had believed that quick solutions for the left ventricle problems would also improve the secondary tricuspid regurgitation (STR). Every active surgeon has been preferred this quick solution in his whole surgery life many times. Medical treatment options aims to improve the underlying disease and the right ventricle failure. TV surgery have proven to yield good outcomes in surgery indicated patients. For patients who are not available for surgery, trans catheter intervention may be an alternative. Due to limited data, the best surgical techniques are still in question, with no clear answer, particularly for STR. Key factor in determining prognosis, timing for intervention and longer-term outcome is the right ventricular function at the time of prognosis.

Keywords: tricuspid valve, annuloplasty, regurgitation, annular ring, De Vega

1. Introduction

In the past, the TV has received less attention than the other heart valves in terms of pathophysiology and surgical treatment. TV is part of a complex functional structure that involves the right atrium (RA), the right ventricle (RV), and the pulmonary artery (PA) circulation. The prevalence of TV disease is steadily increasing, with the tricuspid regurgitation (TR), the most common form, occurring in an estimated 65–85% of the European population [1]. The most common type of TV disease is functional tricuspid regurgitation (FTR), occurring secondary to the dilation of the tricuspid annulus and/or the tethering of the valve leaflets due to RV dilation and dysfunction. However, with the recent increase in right-sided implantation of transvenous devices (pacemakers, implantable defibrillators), there has been a parallel increase in the risk of organic tricuspid disease. Recent data suggests that TR is not benign, and many patients would benefit from intervention during left-sided valve surgery or in the early period of isolated TV disease (TVD) [2]. The clinical evaluation of TVD is often difficult because of a lack of early clinical characteristics, as the disease might progress when it is diagnosed by a consultant. In order to manage symptoms, prevent complications, and improve quality of life, advanced TVD has to be surgically repaired or replaced [3].

Isolated TR patients are rarely referred for valve surgery and most repairs are performed at the same time with other planned cardiac procedures. With an in-hospital mortality rate up to 37% re-operations for evident TR and heart valve disease or for recurrent TR, generally they are not routinely recommended for most

IntechOpen

patients [2]. The current American and European guidelines advocate a more proactive approach for the treatment of TR and/or annular dilatation during left-sided valve surgery. For its better superior long-term outcomes, tricuspid annuloplasty is the preferred technique. This renewed interest in surgical repair has been fueled by the development of a new generation of tricuspid annuloplasty rings and the technological advances in transcatheter treatment, which has expanded to include tricuspid pathologies in otherwise inoperable patients with advanced tricuspid disease and cardiomyopathy. Aggressive approach to surgical treatment is more widely adopted, rather than prophylactic interventions. Still, aggressive tricuspid surgery remains an area of controversy, while surgical repair is considered the gold standard for functional TR [4]. An important note is that presumably because of right ventricle anatomy the pathophysiology of functional TR is understood much less than functional mitral regurgitation (MR). Besides, the left ventricle function has a key role for the function of the right ventricle [5].

2. Anatomy and physiology

The heart has four functional valves and TV is the largest one, with a normal orifice area between 7–9 cm^2 (**Figure 1**) [6], apically located. Due to the low pressure differences between the RA and the RV, the large size of the TV can function at low gradient (<2 mm Hg) and low peak transtricuspid diastolic velocities [6]. The leaflets, the papillary muscles, the chordal attachments, and the annulus (with attached atrium and ventricle) are the components of the TV [7]. The integrity and harmony of these components result successful valve function.

2.1 The leaflets

TV closure during systole needs the normal function of the leaflets and their relationship with chordae and papillary muscle, although they are also closely related to the size and function of RV. RV pressure overload and remodeling was associated with up to 49% increase in TV leaflet size compared to controls in recent screenings, and when this increase in size was insufficient to cover the tricuspid valve closure area, there was a gradual increase in TR severity. observed [8]. The TV typically consists of 3 leaflets of unequal size. Healthy subjects may have anatomical

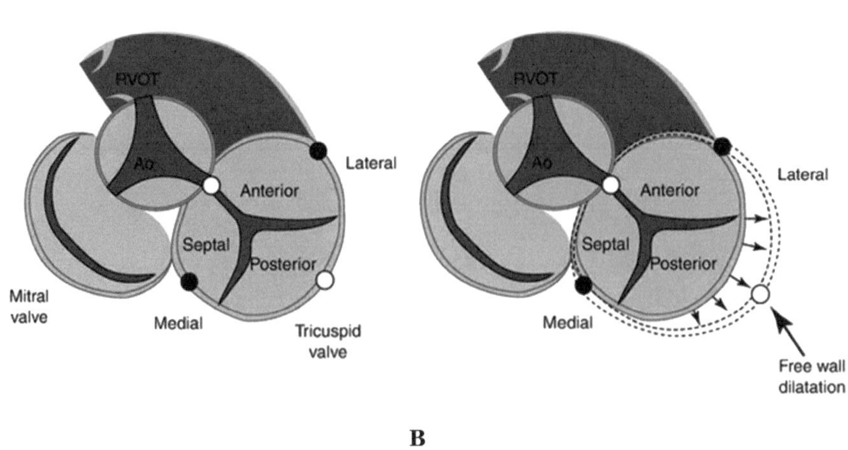

Figure 1.
A) Tricuspid valve and rhe relations with the other valves. B) The weak sies of the tricuspid aparatus with tendency for dilation.

variants consisting of 2 (bicuspid) leaflets or more than 3 leaflets [9]. Definition according to their anatomical positions in the body, these 3 leaflets would be septal, anterior-superior, and inferior: called septal, anterior, and posterior leaflets [10]. The anterior leaflet is the largest, whereas the posterior leaflet is notable for the presence of multiple scallops. The septal leaflet is the smallest and arises medially, directly from the tricuspid annulus above the interventricular septum. It is attached to the tricuspid annulus directly above the interventricular septum [11]. The anatomical markings for each leaflet vary considerably based on the size and shape of the annulus; still, the commissure between the septal and posterior leaflets is often prominent, located near coronary sinus entrance into the right atrium (**Figure 2**).

When we examine the integrity of the four heart valves the noncoronary sinus of valsalva of aortic root is typically adjacent to commissure between the septal and anterior leaflets: the anteroseptal commissure. This is the longest commissure, as the anterior and septal leaflets are often the longest circumferentially. The coaptation of the TV is typically at or just below the level of the annulus with a coaptation length of 5–10 mm [12]. This coaptation length is the potential reserve for keeping the function of the TV when right side of the heart is affected as dilation.

2.2 Chordae and papillary muscles

Tensor apparatus of TV are the papillary muscles and chordae. The posterior and septal leaflets supported by medial papillary muscle group cordae and anterior and posterior leaflets supported by anterior papillary muscle group cordae [6].

The accessory chordae may protrude from the right ventricular free wall or the moderator band. Hence, the septal and anterior leaflets of the TV are attached to the interventricular septum, and the anterior and posterior leaflets are attached to a

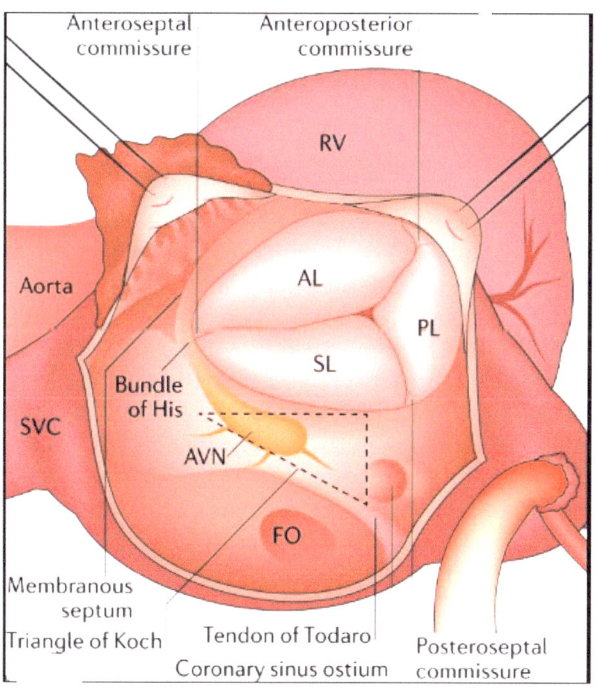

Figure 2.
The schematic seen of the Tricuspid Valve and the relation of heart conduction system (AVN: AN node, SVC: Superior Vena Cava, FO: Fossa Ovalis (Also this is the key anatomic tissue for trans septal mitral valve intervention), RV: Right Ventricle).

large anterior papillary muscle along the anterolateral right ventricular wall. Due to the fixed length of the chordae, the displacement of septal or lateral wall positions of the RV would affect tricuspid leaflet coaptation. Therefore, tricuspid annular sizing algorithms have been based on the dimension of the base of the septal leaflet [13]. The number of chordae varied from 17 to 36 with an average of 25 chordae [7]. Since the septal leaflets that is fixed to the septal wall is quite immobile, there is little space for the free wall of the right ventricle/tricuspid annulus to expand (**Figure 1**) [14].

Transcatheter interventions of the heart, the chordae can interact with catheters and interventional devices, causing additional difficulty during transcatheter approaches for TV. Besides, the mechanical properties and superstructure of the TV chordae tendineae in normal humans are composed of somewhat flat collagen bundles made of collagen fibrin matrices, with less extensibility than normal mitral valve chordae of comparable size [15].

2.3 Tricuspid valve annulus

The TV is situated within an elliptical, nonplanar annulus. The normal tricuspid ring is D-shaped, non-planar with two distinct segments: a larger C-shaped segment corresponding to the free wall of the RA and RV, and a shorter, relatively straighter segment corresponding to the septal leaflet and the ventricular septum [7]. Flexible fibroadipose tissue is the composition the annular ring. During the cardiac cycle composition of the annulus allows geometrical changes, it is rounder during diastole, and during systole it becomes more elliptical by the interventricular septum bulges into the RV [16]. The tricuspid annulus has a complex, three-dimensional structure that differs from the more symmetrical "saddle-shaped" mitral ring. This shape has implications for the design and implementation of new annuloplasty rings, rather than the existing planar annuloplasty rings in the tricuspid position [11]. Fukuda et al. conducted a real-time, three-dimensional transthoracic echocardiographic research and examined 15 healthy subjects and 16 patients with functional TR (12/16 had moderate to severe TR). They mapped the tricuspid annulus throughout the cardiac cycle and reconstructed it using a computer workstation. The healthy subjects had a non-planar, elliptical tricuspid annulus, with the posteroseptal segment being the lowest relative to the right ventricular apex and the anteroseptal segment being the highest. Patients with functional TR often had rather planar annulus compared to the elliptical shape in healthy subjects; the latter mainly expanded in the septal-lateral direction (F resulting in a more circular shape. The authors concluded that novel approaches or rings tailored to the unique shape of the tricuspid ring could improve ventricular function and reduce leaflet stress [17].

The tricuspid annulus is a dynamic structure that can produce significant changes (up to ~30%) in the area it creates during the cardiac cycle. It is greater in end-systolic/early diastole and during atrial systole, as well as under loading conditions [6]. When measured in healthy subjects using 3D echocardiography, the normal tricuspid annulus has a circumference of 12 ± 1 cm and an area of 11 ± 2 cm^2 [17]. During surgery it is more difficult to identify the TV annulus when it compared with the mitral valve annulus. The posteroseptal tricuspid annulus is more ventricular, but anteroseptal portion is more atrial [18].

3. Cause, diagnosis, and natural history

Two forms of TR are primary and secondary. Primary TR is seen less and can be the congenital or acquired disease processes that affect the leaflets or chordal structures, or both. Secondary or functional TR (STR or FTR) is more common and secondary to other diseases like left-side heart diseases, pulmonary hypertension, RV dilation, and dysfunction from any cause, without intrinsic lesion of the TV itself. Enlargement of the valve annulus and the right ventricle is the main reason of the STR, any cause of left heart dysfunction or disease of myocardial or valvular causes, RV volume and pressure overload, and dilation of cardiac chambers can be the reason. Less common causes of tricuspid valve pathology include rheumatic, congenital, or other causes (endocarditis, leaflet tear/prolapse, chordal rupture, papillary muscle rupture, or myxomatous degeneration of the tricuspid valve) [19].

3.1 Classification of tricuspid regurgitation

See **Table 1**.

3.1.1 Primary tricuspid regurgitation

Primary TR is seen less than the secondary form may be congenital (Ebstein's anomaly) or acquired diseases of the TV (myxomatous degeneration of the tricuspid valve, leading to TV prolapse, endocarditis, carcinoid syndrome, rheumatic disease, radiation, or trauma). The latter is crucial for patient selection and clinical decision-making, so the two must be differentiated. One of the only causes of TR is that the leads of a pacemaker or defibrillator that pass from the RA to the RV can directly affect the leaflet coaptation. This has been reported in case reports and small series, but might be more important and common than currently detected. In a 2008 publication, by Kim et al. researched the effect of a transtricuspid permanent pacemaker or implantable cardiac defibrillator in 248 subjects using echocardiograms before and after device implantation. The authors found grade 1 or greater worsening of TR after implant in 24.2% of the subjects, and TR worsening was more common in implantable cardiac defibrillators than in permanent pacemakers with mild or lower TR at baseline [20]. The current guidelines do not recommended removal in patients with TR and transtricuspid pacing leads due to the potential to damage the valve and result in serious conditions [21].

3.1.2 Secondary (functional) tricuspid regurgitation

The most common cause of TR is secondary or "functional" insufficiency. STR can be categorized based on the underlying cause or the morphological abnormality of the tricuspid apparatus; some morphologies are clearly associated with specific underlying diseases:

1. STR due to left-sided heart disease (valve disease or left ventricular dysfunction),

2. STR due to any cause of pulmonary arterial hypertension (chronic lung disease, pulmonary thromboembolism, left-to-right shunt disease, or systolic

Primary	Secondary
Rheumatic Infective endocarditis Iatrogenic (device leads, endomyocardial biopsy) Congenital (eg, Ebstein's, levo-transposition of the great arteries) Other (eg, trauma, carcinoid, drugs, irradiation)	Pulmonary hypertension with RV remodeling (primary or secondary to left-sided heart disease) Dilated cardiomyopathy Annular dilation (associated with AF) RV volume overload (shunts/high output)

Table 1.
Tricuspid regurgitation classification table.

pulmonary artery pressure estimated by Doppler >50 mm Hg with no identifiable clinical cause),

3. STR due to any RV dysfunction (myocardial disease or RV ischemia/infarction),

4. STR with no detectable cause of TR (idiopathic STR).

Some morphological abnormalities associated with STR may co-occur, including:

1. tricuspid leaflet attachment or tenting,

2. displacement of papillary muscles,

3. RV dysfunction,

4. enlargement of the annulus and/or RA.

Several studies have concluded that atrial fibrillation (AF), ischemic heart disease associated with mitral regurgitation, rheumatic heart disease, and a large left atrium are associated risk factors of TR [22].

Many factors as preload, afterload, myocardial wall thickness and contractility which can limited by the intact pericardium are determining the right ventricle ejection fraction and the stroke volume. The RV Wall thickness is about 3–4 mm and the mass is approximately six times less than the LV. The RV is adapted to eject blood against a lower pulmonary vascular resistance. RV is low pressure highly compliant cardiac chamber because of low afterload results in reduced wall tension and characterises RV physiology. Before progressive RV dilatation, dysfunction and

Stage	Definition	Valve hemodynamics	Hemodynamic consequences	Clinical symptoms and presentation
B	Progressive TR	Central jet <50% RA Vena contracta width <0.7 cm ERO <0.40 cm^2 Regurgitant volume <45 mL	None	None
C	Asymptomatic severe TR	Central jet ≥50% RA Vena contracta width ≥0.7 cm ERO ≥0.40 cm^2 Regurgitant volume ≥45 mL Dense continuous wave signal with triangular shape Hepatic vein systolic flow reversal	Dilated RV and RA Elevated RA with "c-V" wave	Elevated venous pressure No symptoms
D	Symptomatic severe TR	Central jet ≥50% RA Vena contracta width ≥0.7 cm ERO ≥0.40 cm^2 Regurgitant volume ≥45 mL Dense continuous wave signal with triangular shape Hepatic vein systolic flow reversal	Dilated RV and RA Elevated RA with "c-V" wave	Elevated venous pressure Dyspnea on exertion, fatigue, ascites, edema

c-V wave indicates systolic positive wave; ERO, effective regurgitant orifice; RA, right atrial; RV, right ventricular; and TR, tricuspid regurgitation [23].

Table 2.
Stages of tricuspid regurgitation (AHA Guidelines).

failure progression RV can tolerate this high volume state for prolonged periods. This may occur with or without the development of pulmonary vasculopathy (from chronic high flow). Cresent shape of the RV changes with chronic volume overload to spherical form till limitation of the pericardial capacity. Ventricular interdependence shifts the ventricular septum leftward. LV filling is impaired further compounding a fall in cardiac output (**Table 2**) [8].

4. Diagnosis of tricuspid regurgitation

According to the 2020 AHA guidelines, TTE can differentiate primary TR (abnormal valve leaflets) from STR (normal valve leaflets) for left ventricular-related valve or myocardial disease. PA systolic pressure can be measured by TEE. Characterization of the severity of TR-related regurgitation is based on an integrative assessment of multiple parameters, as recommended by the American Society of Echocardiography and European Association of Echocardiography, but many limitations still remain. In patients with TR undergoing left-heart valve surgery, an annular diastolic diameter >40 mm (or >21 mm/m^2) indicates an increased risk of permanent or progressive TR after isolated mitral valve surgery. PA systolic pressure is estimated from maximal TR velocity. TR velocity for evaluation of RV systolic function is challenged by variation in RV loading condition as well as geometric and image acquisition constraints. Normal RV systolic function is defined by various parameters, including tricuspid annular plane systolic excursion (TAPSE) >16 mm, TV systolic. Other imaging modalities, such as magnetic resonance imaging and CT scanning, can provide more accurate information about the status of the RV [23].

Again according to the AHA guidelines invasive measurement of cardiac index, right–sided diastolic pressures, pulmonary artery pressures, and pulmonary artery pressures and pulmonary vascular resistance, as well as right ventriculography, can be useful when clinical and noninvasive are discordant or inadequate in patients with TR [23].

While TR is one of the main right-sided pathologies that cause right heart failure (RHF), tricuspid stenosis (TS) is a rare etiology for RHF. The increased volume load induces cardiac dilatation, thereby stretching the walls of the cardiac chambers, causing dilation of the tricuspid annulus and enhance the regurgitation of the blood. Therefore, as RHF increases over time, the progressive deterioration of TV functions becomes trapped in a vicious cycle that advances the heart failure. Signs of this pathological mechanism can be seen on echocardiography, and patients with severe TR have right heart enlargement. Other signs observed may include enlargement or pulsation of the inferior vena cava and/or hepatic veins. In addition, the TAPSE can be measured to detect subtle ventricular dysfunction: TAPSE < 8.5 mm is associated with right ventricular ejection fraction less than 25%. If RHF is suspected, investigations including electrocardiogram, natriuretic peptides, and echocardiogram are used to confirm the diagnosis [24].

Echocardiography is routinely used in clinical practice to assess the severity of TR. This includes color doppler flow mapping in at least 2 orthogonal planes, assessment of vena contracta width, flow convergence calculations, and the direction and size of the jet. In addition, the morphology of continuous wave doppler recordings across the valve and pulsed wave doppler of the hepatic veins can be used [25]. Serial evaluations of TR should be interpreted in the clinical context of the patient because, as with functional mitral regurgitation, severity volume status and afterload may be affected by many factors such as The RV shape is complex compared to the left ventricle, appearing as a crescent in cross-section and triangular when viewed from the side [26].

COR	LOE	Recommendations
1	B-NR	1. In patients with severe TR (Stages C and D) undergoing left-sided valve surgery, tricuspid valve surgery is recommended.
2a	B-NR	2. In patients with progressive TR (Stage B) undergoing left-sided valve surgery, tricuspid valve surgery can be beneficial in the context of either 1) tricuspid annular dilation (tricuspid annulus end diastolic diameter >4.0 cm) or 2) prior signs and symptoms of right-sided HF.
2a	B-NR	3. In patients with signs and symptoms of right-sided HF and severe primary TR (Stage D), isolated tricuspid valve surgery can be beneficial to reduce symptoms and recurrent hospitalizations.
2a	B-NR	4. In patients with signs and symptoms of right-sided HF and severe isolated secondary TR attributable to annular dilation (in the absence of pulmonary hypertension or left-sided disease) who are poorly responsive to medical therapy (Stage D), isolated tricuspid valve surgery can be beneficial to reduce symptoms and recurrent hospitalizations.
2b	C-LD	5. In asymptomatic patients with severe primary TR (Stage C) and progressive RV dilation or systolic dysfunction, isolated tricuspid valve surgery may be considered.
2b	B-NR	6. In patients with signs and symptoms of right-sided HF and severe TR (Stage D) who have undergone previous left-sided valve surgery, reoperation with isolated tricuspid valve surgery may be considered in the absence of severe pulmonary hypertension or severe RV systolic dysfunction.

Table 3.
2020 ACC/AHA guideline for the management of patients with valvular heart.

Disease recommendations for intervention timing for TR intervention (Level A: High quality evidence from more than 1 rondomised clinical trial (RCT) or meta-analyses of high –quality RCTs or one or more RCTs corroborated by high-quality registry studies. Level B-R: Moderate-quality evidence from 1 or more RCT sor meta-analyses of moderate-quality RCTs. Level B-NR: moderate –quality evidence from 1 or more well-designed, well-executed nonrandomized studies observational studies, or registry studies or meta-analysis of such studies. Level C-LD: Randomized or nonrandomized observational or registry studies with limitations of design or execution or meta-analyses of such studies or physiological or mechanistic studies in human subjects. Level C-EO: Consensus of expert opinion based on clinical experience.) (**Table 3**) [23].

By using experimental models it has been estimated that left ventricle contractions contribute 20% to 40% of RV systolic pressure and volume output [27]. And also both two ventricles share same biochemical environment, by this way any systemic and local neurohormonal parameters result in improvements in biventricular function. Importantly, left-sided heart failure with chamber enlargement and mitral regurgitation can cause right-sided pressure overload, RV dilation, tricuspid annulus enlargement, and resultant TR. This mechanical step initially led to the concept that surgical or medical treatment of the left-sided abnormality would result in secondary recovery or improvement in TR. Although there is improvement in TR, this is not always the case [11]. Dreyfus et al have shown that a paradigm advocating treatment of only the proposed "primary" lesion, such as mitral valve disease, will not directly correct tricuspid annular dilation or improve right ventricular function, which are key determinants of functional TR. In their study, the TV annulus was evaluated visually in 311 patients who underwent mitral valve repair between 1989 and 2001. Tricuspid annuloplasty was performed selectively only in patients with twice the tricuspid annular diameter (as measured from anteroseptal commissure to anteroposterior). New York Heart Association class were significantly improved in those who underwent TV annuloplasty. In-hospital mortality and actuarial survival rate were similarly improved in patients undergoing TV annuloplasty, supporting the notion that TV annuloplasty improves patient outcomes during mitral valve repair [18].

In 2020 report by Tirone [28] for degenerative MR they found no correlation between tricuspid annulus of ≥ 40 mm on the development of postoperative TR following mitral valve repair. They concluded that a preoperative echocardiographic diameter of tricuspid annulus ≥ 40 mm is not associated with the development postoperative TR after mitral valve repair for degenerative MR. Furthermore, in their report of extended outcomes of mitral valve repair for degenerative MR, they found that patients were only 2.5% likely to develop severe TR at 20 years after surgery, but the probability increased to 20.8% when moderate-intensity TR was added. It was also very disturbing to find an accumulated new incidence of atrial fibrillation of 32.4% over 20 years. The development of these two adverse events was not associated with repeat MR and may have been interdependent. The reporter recommends that tricuspid annuloplasty should be performed during mitral valve surgery when there is moderate or severe tricuspid regurgitation and in patients with atrial fibrillation or a dilated right ventricular cavity (systolic diameter ≥30 mm), even in the absence of significant tricuspid regurgitation [18, 29].

5. Current surgical approaches to tricuspid regurgitation

In the past decades, intervention was believed to be unnecessary, as repairing secondary TR would resolve the problems in the left ventricle, which was thought to help TR regress as well. The first experience regarding the prognosis of FTR was reported by Braunwald in 1967. Braunwald claimed that untreated FTR naturally resolves after treating mitral valve disease [30]. Later, Carpentier recommended surgical intervention for FTR in patients with mitral valve disease [31]. However, today's understanding suggests aggressive intervention to resolve this disease. Repairing left-sided valve disease has resulted in increased survival rates, making the long-term sequelae of TR more pronounced. During left heart surgery, severe secondary TR should also be corrected. In cases of moderate or even lower right ventricular dysfunction or enlarged tricuspid valve annulus TR should be addressed as well [32]. The indications for tricuspid valve procedure during left heart valve surgery are relatively simple, though there is limited data on how to approach a patient with functional TR with no indications for left heart surgery. The preferred approach for these patients has not been well defined [33]. The main surgical technique to repair functional TR with a dilated ring and normal leaflet and chordal structures is by rigid or flexible annular open or closed rings, which are also used in mitral valve surgery, aiming to reduce annulus size and provide leaflet coaptation [11].

Contrary to findings regarding isolated TV surgery, the increased risk of mortality associated with concomitant tricuspid annuloplasty during mitral valve surgery seems almost negligible in current practice. TV repair takes an additional 15 to 20 minutes, but it can be performed without prolonging the CPB time by removing the cross-clamp in the working and perfused heart. The incidence of heart block requiring pacemaker implantation is potentially greater with concurrent tricuspid surgery, although this has been refused by most comparative series, seeming largely dependent on the preferred annuloplasty technique. Similarly, the current literature has yet to confirm the theoretical incremental risk of postoperative bleeding with the addition of a right atriotomy suture line [34].

The anatomical characteristics of the TV determine the repair technique:

1. Annulus intervention (annuloplasty),
2. Leaflets (e.g., triangular resection),
3. Chordae (e.g., transfers or new chordae),
4. Papillary muscles (e.g., sliding technique).

5.1 Annuloplasty

Despite the multiple repair strategies for TV, the ring annuloplasty technique is the preferred treatment for preventing the long-term recurrence of TR associated with suture annuloplasty [35, 36]. Tricuspid annuloplasty devices, whether rigid or incomplete semirigid rings for creating annular remodeling, or flexible bands that provide annular reduction, are often focused on restructuring annular movement. To date, there has been no clear evidence of superiority for any annuloplasty device for preventing the recurrence of TR [37]. In functional or secondary TR, the non-planar native tricuspid annulus is larger, flatter, and more circular. Hence, the ideal annuloplasty device should consider the geometric changes and restore the normal three-dimensional elliptical shape of the tricuspid annulus to reduce leaflet stress and tethering It should also focus on remodeling along the right ventricular free wall, but have an open design to protect the transmission system. Ideally, such a device would be "resilient" in areas of three-dimensional motion or areas prone to ring separation, particularly along the membranous septum [38].

5.1.1 Kay annuloplasty

The first type of annuloplasty is suture annuloplasty, which can be done in one of two ways [39]. First Kay annuloplasty was introduced in 1962: involves creating a functional bicuspid valve by placing a suture through the posterior leaflet's commissure [40]. This surgical technique places a pledget-supported bed suture from the anterior-posterior commissure through the posterior annulus to the posteroseptal commissure. Deloche et al. have demonstrated posterior annular dilatation in functional TR, suggesting that this method would work in selected cases [41]. In 1965 Herald Kay reported his Kay bicuspidization procedure, where the posterior leaflet is plicated along the annulus, has shown good mid-term and long-term results [40]. Ghanta et al. have modified this technique (**Figure 3**) [42].

5.1.2 DeVega annuloplasty

DeVega annuloplasty was introduced in 1972 as an alternative [43]. The classical De Vega annuloplasty consists of a pair of continuous sutures, running along the anterior and posterior annulus, often corresponding to the free walls of the right ventricle. The septal part of the annulus is typically not involved in the expansion and is reserved to protect the transmission system. In the classical De Vega technique, a 2/0 or 3/0 polypropylene suture starts from the posterior end of the septal part of the annulus and continues counterclockwise in the posterior and anterior parts. The suture needle is inserted 1 to 2 mm deep, into 5 to 6 mm long knots. When the suture reaches the fibrous trigone, the anteroseptal commissure

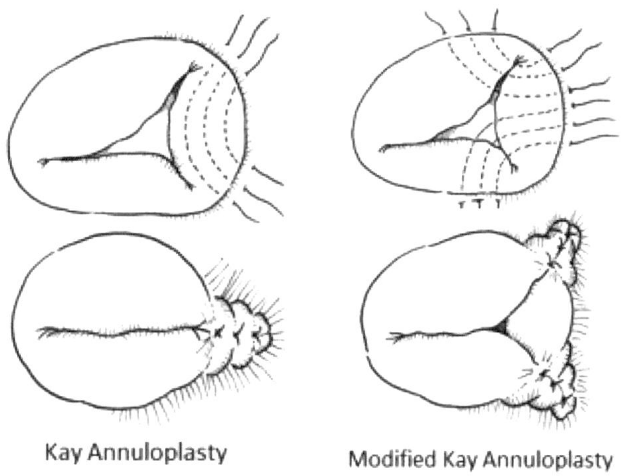

Figure 3.
The original and modified technique of Kay annulopasty.

is inverted on a teflon felt pledget; in the second suture, each knot of the ring interposes with that of the first. The suture ends where it starts, and a teflon felt is attached to the pledget. The degree of narrowing of the annulus can be measured from 25 to 29 mm using a mechanical valve sizer or Hegar dilator, depending on the patient's body surface area. Note that mild stenosis is better tolerated than regurgitation. When performed routinely, the valve can be tested by injecting cold saline into the right ventricle using a bulb syringe (**Figure 4**) [44].

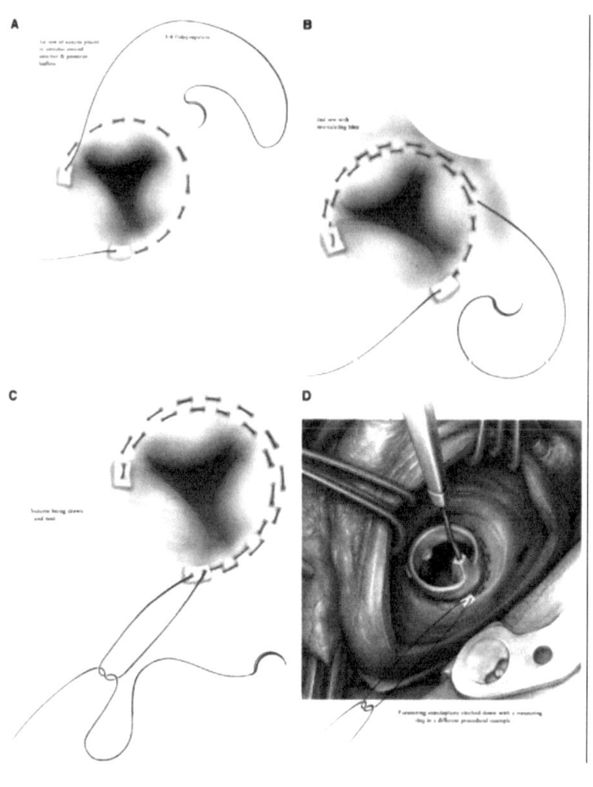

Figure 4.
De Vega Annuloplasty.

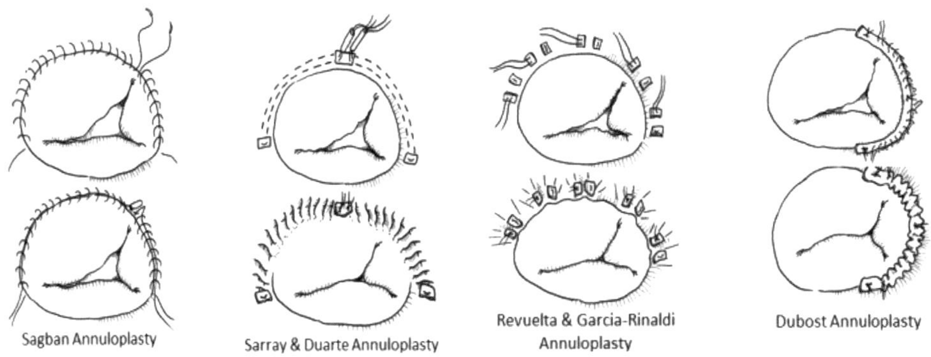

Figure 5.
The several modified techniques of De Vega annuloplasty.

As a result of gliding effect recurrent TR secondary to Bowstring phenomenon is seen after classical De Vega annuloplasty often in the setting of moderate to severe regurgitation. There are several modifications of classical De Vega annuloplasty for example, Revuelta and Garcia-Rinaldi, Dubost, Sagban, and Sarray and Duarte (**Figure 5**) [45].

5.1.3 Carpentier ring annuloplasty

The next technique is ring annuloplasty, introduced by Carpentier in 1971. This is where a rigid or semirigid ring is introduced to control the dilatation of the annulus [39].

A rare complication that deserves focus is injury to the right coronary artery (RCA). Plications caused by aggressive reduction of the tricuspid annulus or deep penetration of purulent string sutures may impair RCA flow [37]. Note that severe arrhythmias, persistent ST elevation on electrocardiogram, or RV dysfunction following cardiopulmonary bypass would affect the RCA. Prompt grafting of the distal RCA or removal of the annuloplasty band is an effective strategy to deal with this rare complication, but early recognition is key for good outcomes [37].

A 2014 meta-analysis compared these techniques and found bicuspidization or the Kay method to be associated with a higher risk of recurrent TR. Still, ring annuloplasty was found to give better results in reducing the risk of recurrence. There was no significant difference in late survival rates, although ring annuloplasty provided significant reduction in early mortality [46]. A more recent 2020 meta-analysis concluded that mortality and TR incidence rates were comparable among ring and suture. Other flexible rings were found to have a higher TR ratio than rigid rings. However, this systematic review excluded articles with primary TR. There is still a limited number of suitable research and a lack of large randomized studies (**Figure 6**) [47].

5.2 Leaflets maneuvers

As described by Castedo et al., other approaches include edge-to-edge repairs, like the Alfieri repair, and DeVega-style purse-string suturing techniques to reduce the anterior and posterior parts of the annulus [48, 49].

There have been some auxiliary techniques to increase ring annuloplasty methods, particularly in leaflet tethering formed by right ventricular dilatation and annulus enlargement. Enlarging the anterior leaflet with a pericardial patch increases leaflet coaptation and provides leaflet mobility (**Figure 7**) [50].

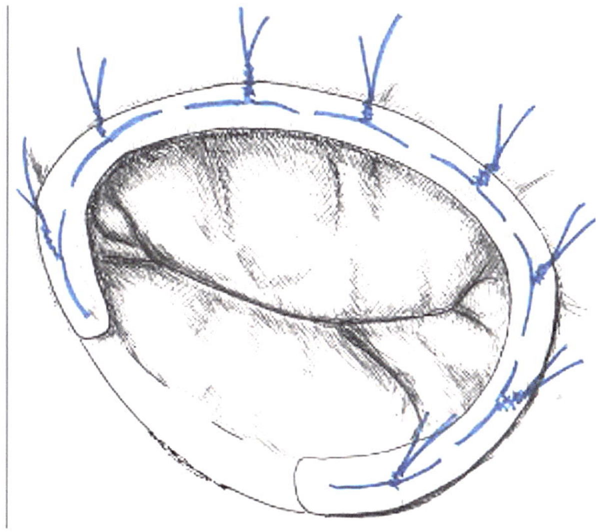

Figure 6.
TV ring annuloplasty.

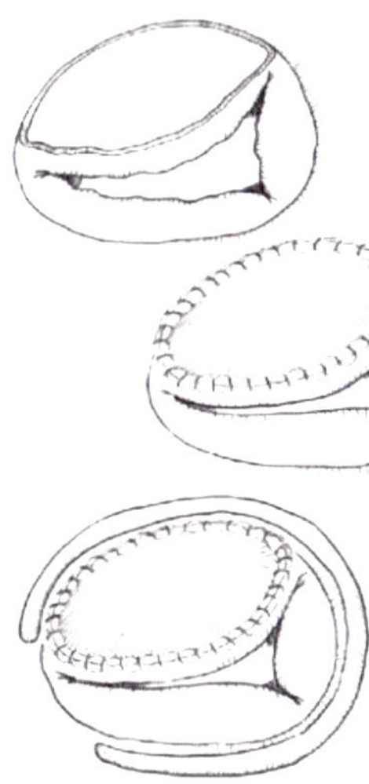

Figure 7.
The anterior leaflet of TV is enlarged by using a pericardial patch.

Double-orifice valve repair is achieved by approximating the free edges of the septal and newly formed anteroposterior leaflets. This is very effective in dealing with complex acquired TR (**Figure 8**) [51].

The 'clover' technique consists of stitching together the middle point of the free edges of the tricuspid leaflets, producing a clover-shaped valve (**Figure 9**) [52].

Combination of some factors like the technique of the operation, decision of annuloplasty type, unrecognized severe leaflet tethering area mismatch between the leaflets and the annuloplasty ring. In cases of severe tethering enlargement of posterior and anterior leaflet can be used. However there is no evidence that this is superior to tricuspid valve replacement [50].

Recurrent TR is probably due to a combination of factors: operative technique, type of annuloplasty used, unrecognized severe tethering of the leaflet, and

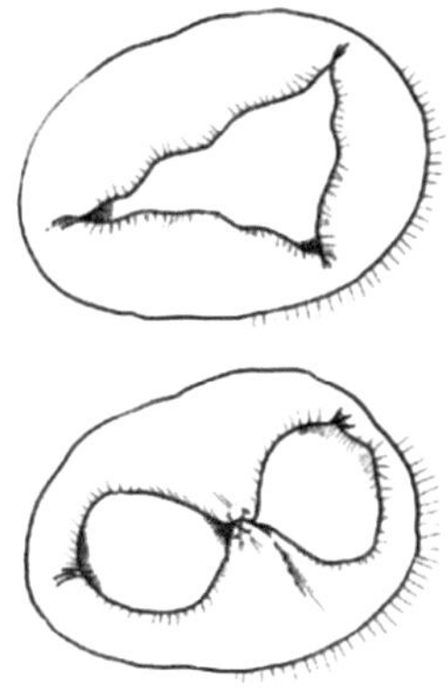

Figure 8.
Double orifice technique like in Alfieri technique.

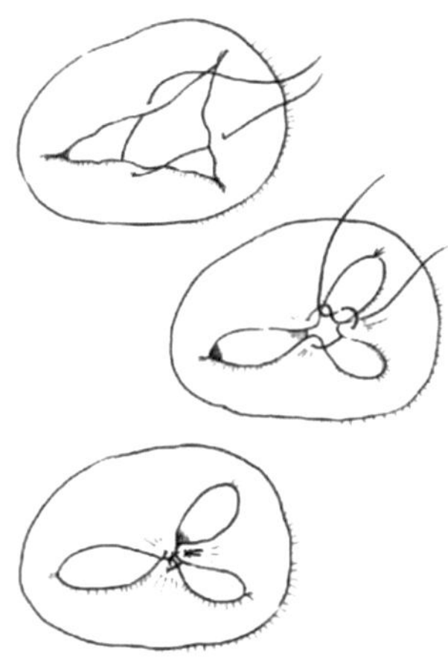

Figure 9.
The stages of clover technique.

mismatch between the area of the leaflets and the area of the annuloplasty ring. Some surgeons advocate patch enlarging the anterior and posterior leaflets in cases of severe tethering but there is no evidence that this is superior to tricuspid valve replacement [50].

6. Discussion

In the absence of concurrent tricuspid valve repair, the incidence of TR after mitral valve surgery is somewhat dependent on the MR mechanism. A US study on 5223 patients reported worse survival rates at a 4-year follow-up of TR, independent of age, right and left ventricular systolic function, or right ventricular diameter. TR has been associated with less survival times in ischemic or non-ischemic cardiomyopathy with or without heart failure symptoms [32, 53]. Matsuyama et al. followed up 174 patients for 8 years and found that only 16% who underwent non-ischemic degenerative mitral valve surgery without tricuspid valve surgery developed 3 to 4 TRs [54]. TR seems much more common in patients who had mitral valve repair due to functional ischemic mitral regurgitation. Matsunaga et al. investigated 70 patients who underwent mitral valve repair due to functional ischemic mitral regurgitation and found that 30% (21/70) had at least moderate TR before surgery. Postoperatively, moderate TR increased by 25% in 1 year, 53% in 1 to 3 years, and 74% at the 3-year follow-up [55].

Even after successful mitral valve repair, significant residual tricuspid valve regurgitation contributes to poor postoperative hemodynamic outcomes. King et al. found high early and late mortality rates in patients who required tricuspid valve surgery after mitral valve operation. The authors encouraged liberal use of tricuspid annuloplasty in the first mitral valve surgery. Surgical series have demonstrated significant improvement in recurrent TR, survival, and event-free survival rates with successful tricuspid valve repair (primarily when combined with other valve surgeries) [56].

Rigid annuloplasty rings appear to have lower TR recurrence rates than DeVega and flexible band annuloplasty [57]. Algarni et al. compared rigid rings with flexible bands in 713 TV annuloplasty patients in 2020. The authors found that the type of TV annuloplasty did not affect survival or tricuspid valve reoperation. However, there was a trend of higher cumulative incidence of recurrent moderate TR with flexible bands compared to rigid rings [58].

Dreyfus et al. suggested that annular dilatation measuring 70 mm or more during mitral valve repair surgery is an indication for annuloplasty, even in the absence of TR. The authors also demonstrated that TR was increased by at least 2 degrees in 45% of patients undergoing isolated mitral valve repair, supporting the perspective that tricuspid dilatation is a progressive process that often warrants preventive surgical treatment [18]. Singh et al. found no difference in survival or need for TV reoperation over 10 years of follow-up with TV repair compared to tricuspid valve replacement in patients with organic TR. Tricuspid valve repair is associated with better perioperative, midterm, and event-free survival rates than TV replacement in patients with organic tricuspid disease. TV replacement demonstrated higher mortality. The authors suggested that the higher perioperative mortality with replacement may be due to a hard object (the tricuspid valve) in a deformable low-pressure cavity (the right ventricle), resulting in right ventricular dysfunction and a low-output state perioperatively. The authors concluded that there was no difference in terms of functional class among the groups, although the patients had fewer recurrent TRs with repair versus replacement (62% versus 95% had mild or less TR at the final echocardiographic follow-up) [2].

Due to the significant risks of isolated tricuspid valve surgery and the poor prognosis of TR, less invasive approaches like robotic or endoscopic methods or innovative approaches like transcatheter have been needed. Currently, their use is not as common as mitral procedures, as the anatomical features of the tricuspid valve and associated apparatuses make TR treatment with minimally invasive surgery and transcatheter treatment more difficult [59, 60]. Even though severe TR is largely associated with mortality, patients with normal ventricular function can live for years, even decades, without the tricuspid valve. Arbulu et al. performed tricuspid vulvectomy without changing the tricuspid valve in patients with infective endocarditis secondary to IV drug addiction. During long-term follow-up, most patients (37 of 55; 67%) did not require TV replacement, and only a small number of patients without TV developed severe and permanent right ventricular dysfunction. Therefore, if there is only one underlying cardiovascular disease responsible for TR, this may be more important in patients with secondary TR [61].

Gursoy et al. reported that female sex, low preoperative functional capacity, low body surface area, enlarged left atrial size, enlarged right ventricular size, and increased square root of left ventricular mass index were effective on functional TR progression. After these parameters were studied in a multivariate logistic regression analysis, only female sex and left atrial size were found to be independent risk factors [62].

The recurrence of significant TR after tricuspid annuloplasty is around 8 to 15% at 1 month after surgery, depending on various factors (e.g., preoperative TR severity, pulmonary hypertension, RV dilation, pacemaker, LV dysfunction, increased LV remodeling, severe tethering of tricuspid leaflets, or the DeVega technique instead of ring annuloplasty). Most of randomized and observational researches have shown that particularly in patients with severe tricuspid annular dilatation or pulmonary hypertension, repair the valve with ring annuloplasty techniques are more durable than suture annuloplasty ones. Long-term survival after tricuspid valve surgery for severe TR is influenced by a variety of preoperative factors like advanced heart failure symptoms, comorbidity, and end-organ dysfunction, rather than the type of surgery or the cause of TR. Ring annuloplasty may be associated with better results compared to the DeVega technique. The results of annuloplasty alone have not always been consistent. This may be associated with the degree of narrowing of the tricuspid opening, among other factors; thus, it has been recommended to reduce the size of the tricuspid annulus to prevent recurrent TR, considering the patient's body size [63].

The ESC 2017 guidelines recommend ring annuloplasty as the preferred modality for STR. Besides, in cases of severe tethering or severe enlargement of the annulus, replacement should be considered. Still, a very recent 2020 meta-analysis found no comparable differences among these techniques. There is still a lack of adequate research on valve interventions in TR, so the most effective intervention has yet to be clarified [64].

7. Conclusion

Intervention for the tricuspid valve disease has entered a new era with evolving guidelines and the development of new surgical annuloplasty devices and techniques, as well as conceptual transcatheter options. Still, the implementation of such novel techniques requires a significant infrastructure and increased costs. The current guidelines now emphasize surgical repair of functional tricuspid regurgitation during left-sided valve intervention, even during the repair of severely enlarged annulus in the absence of significant tricuspid regurgitation. The newly developed annular rings have been redesigned to protect the transmission system from adverse effects and to better mimic or preserve the normal tricuspid geometry. Finally, there is now an increasing early experience with new transcatheter approaches for managing very high-risk patients with advanced tricuspid valve disease. Regarding repair, the findings tend to increasingly favor rings, and among these, rigid rings that preserve the geometry.

According to our opinion, as mentioned above, it is very clear that if the patient has a severe TR, it is not true to left it as it is. If the patient has operation indication due to mitral valve disease, transseptal approach from right atrium with bicaval cannulation will be helpful for both valve intervention. By this way the surgeon consider to minimize the aortic cross clamp time. However which technique will be chosen is up to the some factors like experience of the surgeon, limitation of the sources, the degree of the regurgitation and the size of the TV annulus and right ventricle. If you don't have any annular ring for plasty, De Vega, Kay annuloplasty techniques or the modifications can be preferable. Also using teflon felt or pericardial patch like a ring is the other choices. In De Vega technique we use the same sizer with the replaced prostetic mitral valve for the reducing tricuspid annulus. If the patient has minimum or moderate TR also this kind of simple or particle techniques also can be preferable. In severe TR, ring annuloplasty has better middle and long term results then the others. Annuloplasty ring sizers can be use or one or double size larger then the prosthetic mitral valve can be used for the TV annular ring. In my opinion after the TV repair testing by saline injection must be done but the result is not certain for the future progress of the valve. Again to our consideration and observation TV intervention with the mitral valve intervention does not effect the early operation mortality and morbidity.

Conflict of interest

The authors declare no conflict of interest.

Author details

Fevzi Sarper Türker[1]*, Zeki Temiztürk[2] and Davut Azboy[3]

1 Istanbul Provincial Directorate of Health, Cardiovascular Surgery Clinic, Mehmet Akif Ersoy Thoracic and Cardiovascular Surgery Training Research Hospital, Turkey

2 Cardiovascular Surgery Clinic, Başakşehir ÇAM and Sakura City Hospital, Turkey

3 Cardiovascular Surgery Clinic, Elaziğ Fethi Sekin City Hospital, Turkey

*Address all correspondence to: sarperturker@gmail.com

References

[1] Arsalan M, Walther T, Smith RL, Grayburn PA. Tricuspid regurgitation diagnosis and treatment. European Heart Journal. 2017;**38**(9):634-638

[2] Singh SK, Tang GH, Maganti MD, Armstrong S, Williams WG, David TE, et al. Midterm outcomes of tricuspid valve repair versus replacement for organic tricuspid disease. The Annals of Thoracic Surgery. 2006;**82**:1735-1741

[3] Harris C, Croce B, Munkholm-Larsen S. Tricuspid valve disease. Annals of Cardiothoracic Surgery. 2017;**6**(3):294-294

[4] El-Eshmawi A, Pandis D, Adams DH, Tang GH. Tricuspid valve surgery: Repair and replacement. Minerva Cardioangiologica. 2018;**66**(6):700-712

[5] Haddad F, Hunt SA, Rosenthal DN, Murphy DJ. Right ventricular function in cardiovascular disease, part I. anatomy, physiology, aging, and functional assessment of the right ventricle. Circulation. 2008;**117**: 1436-1448

[6] Hahn RT. State-of-the-art review of echocardiographic imaging in the evaluation and treatment of functional tricuspid regurgitation. Circulation. Cardiovascular Imaging. 2016;**9**(12): e005332

[7] Dahou A, Levin D, Reisman M, Hahn RT. Anatomy and physiology of the tricuspid valve. JACC: Cardiovascular Imaging. 2019;**12**(3): 458-468

[8] Rana BS, Robinson S, Francis R, Toshner M, Swaans MJ, Agarwal S, et al. Tricuspid regurgitation and the right ventricle in risk stratification and timing of intervention. Echo Research and Practice. 2019;**6**(1):R25-R39

[9] Xanthos T, Dalivigkas I, Ekmektzoglou KA. Anatomic variations of the cardiac valves and papillary muscles of the right heart. Italian Journal of Anatomy and Embryology. 2011;**116**:111-126

[10] Martinez RM, O'Leary PW, Anderson RH. Anatomy and echocardiography of the normal and abnormal tricuspid valve. Cardiology. 2006;**16**:4-11

[11] Rogers JH, Bolling SF. The tricuspid valve: Current perspective and evolving management of tricuspid regurgitation. Circulation. 2009;**119**(20):2718-2725

[12] Silver MD, Lam JHC, Ranganathan N, Wigle ED. Morphology of the human tricuspid valve. Circulation. 1971;**43**:333-348

[13] Yiwu L, Yingchun C, Jianqun Z, Bin Y, Ping B. Exact quantitative selective annuloplasty of the tricuspid valve. The Journal of Thoracic and Cardiovascular Surgery. 2001;**122**: 611-614

[14] Ewy G. Tricuspid valve disease. In: Alpert JS, Dalen JE, Rahimtoola SH, editors. Valvular Heart Disease. 3rd ed. Philadelphia, PA: Lippincott Williams &Wilkins; 2000. pp. 377-392

[15] Lim KO. Mechanical properties and ultrastructure of normal human tricuspid valve chordae tendineae. The Japanese Journal of Physiology. 1980;**30**:455-464

[16] Lau RP, Fishbein GA, Fishbein MC. Specific anatomic considerations for tricuspid interventions. Current Cardiology Reports. 2019;**21**(7):63

[17] Fukuda S, Saracino G, Matsumura Y, Daimon M, Tran H, Greenberg NL, et al. Three-dimensional geometry of the tricuspid annulus in healthy subjects and in patients with functional tricuspid regurgitation: A real-time,

3-dimensional echocardiographic study. Circulation. 2006;**114**(Suppl. 1):492-498

[18] Dreyfus GD, Corbi PJ, Chan KM, Bahrami T. Secondary tricuspid regurgitation or dilation: Which should be the criteria for surgical repair? The Annals of Thoracic Surgery. 2005;**79**:127-132

[19] Cohn LH. Tricuspid regurgitation secondary to mitral valve disease: When and how to repair. Journal of Cardiac Surgery. 1994;**9**:237-241

[20] Kim JB, Spevack DM, Tunick PA, Bullinga JR, Kronzon I, Chinitz LA, et al. The effect of transvenous pacemaker and implantable cardioverter defibrillator lead placement on tricuspid valve function: An observational study. Journal of the American Society of Echocardiography. 2008;**21**:284-287

[21] Love CJ, Wilkoff BL, Byrd CL, Belott PH, Brinker JA, Fearnot NE, et al. Recommendations for extraction of chronically implanted transvenous pacing and defibrillator leads: Indications, facilities, training: North American Society of Pacing and Electrophysiology Lead Extraction Conference Faculty. Pacing and Clinical Electrophysiology. 2000;**23**:544-551

[22] Shiran A, Najjar R, Adawi S, Aronson D. Risk factors for progression of functional tricuspid regurgitation. The American Journal of Cardiology. 2014;**113**(6):995-1000

[23] Otto CM, Nishimura RA, Bonow RO, Carabello BA, Erwin JP 3rd, Gentile F, et al. 2020 ACC/AHA Guideline for the Management of Patients With Valvular Heart Disease: Executive Summary: A Report of the American College of Cardiology/American Heart Association Joint Committee on Clinical Practice Guidelines. Circulation. 2021;**143**(5):e228

[24] Yoganathan A, Khan SNM, Khan H, Thirunavukarasu SA, Elghanam MA, Harky A. Tricuspid valve diseases: Interventions on the forgotten heart valve. Journal of Cardiac Surgery. 2021;**36**(1):219-228

[25] Zoghbi WA, Enriquez-Sarano M, Foster E, Grayburn PA, Kraft CD, Levine RA, et al. Recommendations for evaluation of the severity of native valvular regurgitation with two dimensional and Doppler echocardiography. Journal of the American Society of Echocardiography. 2003;**16**:777-802

[26] Lorenz CH, Walker ES, Morgan VL, Klein SS, Graham TP Jr. Normal human right and left ventricular mass, systolic function, and gender differences by cine magnetic resonance imaging. Journal of Cardiovascular Magnetic Resonance. 1999;**1**:7-21

[27] Suga H, Sagawa K, Shoukas AA. Load independence of the instantaneous pressure-volume ratio of the canine left ventricle and effects of epinephrine and heart rate on the ratio. Circulation Research. 1973;**32**:314-322

[28] David TE. Tricuspid valve annuloplasty at the time of mitral valve surgery: Is it justified in all cases? Indian Journal of Thoracic Cardiovascular Surgery. 2020;**36**(2):88-90

[29] David TE, David CM, Tsang W, Lafreniere-Roula M, Manlhiot C. Long-term results of mitral valve repair for regurgitation due to leaflet prolapse. Journal of the American College of Cardiology. 2019;**74**:1044-1053

[30] Braunwald NS, Ross J Jr, Morrow AG. Conservative management of tricuspid regurgitation in patients undergoing mitral valve replacement. Circulation. 1967;**35**(4 suppl):I63-I69

[31] Carpentier A, Deloche A, Hanania G, Forman J, Sellier P, Piwnica A, et al. Surgical management of acquired tricuspid valve disease. The

Journal of Thoracic and Cardiovascular Surgery. 1974;**67**:53-65

[32] Raman SV, Sparks EA, Boudoulas H, Wooley CF. Tricuspid valve disease: Tricuspid valve complex perspective. Current Problems in Cardiology. 2002;**27**(3):103-142

[33] Boudoulas KD, Barbetseas J, Pitsis AA, Boudoulas H. Tricuspid valve disease: The "Forgotten Valve". Cardiology. 2019;**142**(4):235-238

[34] Reich DL, Fischer GW. Perioperative Transesophageal Echocardiography Book. First ed. United States: Elsevier; 2014

[35] Tang GHL, David TE, Singh SK, et al. Tricuspid valve repair with an annuloplasty ring results in improved long-term outcomes. Circulation. 2006;**114**:577-581

[36] McCarthy PM, Bhudia SK, Rajeswaran J, et al. Tricuspid valve repair: Durability and risk factors for failure. The Journal of Thoracic and Cardiovascular Surgery. 2004;**127**:674-685

[37] El-Eshmawi A, Tang GH, Verma S, Yanagawa B, Ruel M, Adams DH. Innovations in tricuspid valve intervention. Current Opinion in Cardiology. 2017;**32**(2):166-173

[38] Pfannmuller B, Doenst T, Eberhardt K, et al. Increased risk of dehiscence after tricuspid valve repair with rigid annuloplasty rings. The Journal of Thoracic and Cardiovascular Surgery. 2012;**143**:1050-1055

[39] Belluschi I, Del Forno B, Lapenna E, et al. Surgical techniques for tricuspid valve disease. Frontiers in Cardiovascular Medicine. 2018;**5**:118

[40] Kay JH, Maselli-Campagna G, Tsuji KK. Surgical treatment of tricuspid insufficiency. Annals of Surgery. 1965;**162**:53-58

[41] Deloche A, Guerinon J, Fabiani JN, Morillo F, Caramanian M, Carpentier A, et al. Anatomical study of rheumatic tricuspid valve diseases: Application to the study of various valvuloplasties. Annales de Chirurgie Thoracique et Cardio-Vasculaire. 1973;**12**:343-349

[42] Raja SG, Dreyfus GD. Surgery for functional tricuspid regurgitation: Current techniques, outcomes and emerging concepts. Expert Review of Cardiovascular Therapy. 2009;**7**:73-84

[43] DeVega NG. La anuloplastia selective, reguable y permanente. Revista Española de Cardiología. 1972;**25**:6-9

[44] Antunes MJ. DeVega Annuloplasty of the tricuspid valve. Thoracic and Cardiovascular Surgery. 2003;**8**(4): 169-176

[45] Van Praet KM, Stamm C, Starck CT, Sündermann S, Meyer A, Montagner M, et al. An overview of surgical treatment modalities and emerging transcatheter interventions in the management of tricuspid valve regurgitation. Expert Review of Cardiovascular Therapy. 2018;**16**(2):75-89

[46] Parolari A, Barili F, Pilozzi A, Pacini D. Ring or suture annuloplasty for tricuspid regurgitation? A meta-analysis review. The Annals of Thoracic Surgery. 2014;**98**(6):2255-2263

[47] Veen KM, Etnel JRG, Quanjel TJM, et al. Outcomes after surgery for functional tricuspid regurgitation: A systematic review and meta- analysis. European Heart Journal. 2019;**3**(1):10-18

[48] Castedo E, Canas A, Cabo RA, Burgos R, Ugarte J. Edge-to-Edge tricuspid repair for redeveloped valve incompetence after DeVega's annuloplasty. The Annals of Thoracic Surgery. 2003;**75**:605-606

[49] Castedo E, Monguio E, Cabo RA, Ugarte J. Edge-to-edge technique for correction of tricuspid valve

regurgitation due to complex lesions. European Journal of Cardio-Thoracic Surgery. 2005;**27**:933-934

[50] Dreyfus GD, Raja SG, John Chan KM. Tricuspid leaflet augmentation to address severe tethering in functional tricuspid regurgitation. European Journal of Cardio-Thoracic Surgery. 2008;**34**:908-910

[51] Maisano F, Lorusso R, Sandrelli L, et al. Valve repair for traumatic tricuspid regurgitation. European Journal of Cardio-Thoracic Surgery. 1996;**10**:867-873

[52] De Bonis M, Lapenna E, La Canna G, et al. A novel technique for correction of severe tricuspid valve regurgitation due to complex lesions. European Journal of Cardio-Thoracic Surgery. 2004;**25**:760-765

[53] Nath J, Foster E, Heidenreich PA. Impact of tricuspid regurgitation on long-term survival. Journal of the American College of Cardiology. 2004;**43**(3):405-409

[54] Matsuyama K, Matsumoto M, Sugita T, Nishizawa J, Tokuda Y, Matsuo T. Predictors of residual tricuspid regurgitation after mitral valve surgery. Annals of Thoracic Surgery. 2003;**75**:1826-1828

[55] Matsunaga A, Duran CM. Progression of tricuspid regurgitation after repaired functional ischemic mitral regurgitation. Circulation. 2005;**112**(suppl):453-457

[56] King RM, Schaff HV, Danielson GK, Gersh BJ, Orszulak TA, Piehler JM, et al. Surgery for tricuspid regurgitation late after mitral valve replacement. Circulation. 1984;**70**(suppl):193-197

[57] Ghanta RK, Chen R, Narayanasamy N, McGurk S, Lipsitz S, Chen FY, et al. Suture bicuspidization of the tricuspid valve versus ring annuloplasty for repair of functional tricuspid regurgitation: Midterm results of 237 consecutive patients. The Journal of Thoracic and Cardiovascular Surgery. 2007;**133**:117-126

[58] Algarni KD, Alfonso J, Pragliola C, Kheirallah H, Adam AI, Arafat AA. Long-term outcomes of tricuspid valve repair: The influence of the annuloplasty prosthesis. The Annals of Thoracic Surgery. 2021;**112**(5):1493-1500

[59] Faletra FF, Leo LA, Paiocchi VL, Schlossbauer SA, Borruso MG, Pedrazzini G, et al. Imaging-based tricuspid valve anatomy by computed tomography, magnetic resonance imaging, two and three-dimensional echocardiography: Correlation with anatomic specimen. European Heart Journal Cardiovascular Imaging. 2019;**20**(1):1-13

[60] Taramasso M, Alessandrini H, Latib A, Asami M, Attinger-Toller A, Biasco L, et al. Outcomes after current transcatheter tricuspid valve intervention. Mid-term results from the International TriValve Registry. JACC. Cardiovascular Interventions. 2019;**12**(2):155-165

[61] Arbulu A, Holmes RJ, Asfaw I. Tricuspid valvulectomy without replacement. Twenty years' experience. The Journal of Thoracic and Cardiovascular Surgery. 1991;**102**(6): 917-922

[62] Gürsoy M, Bakuy V, Hatemi AC, Bulut G, Kılıçkesmez K, İnce N, et al. Long-term prognosis of mild functional tricuspid regurgitation after mitral valve replacement. Anadolu Kardiyoloji Dergisi. 2014;**14**(1):34-39. DOI: 10.5152/ akd.2013.239

[63] Selke FW, Ruel M. Atlas of Cardiac Surgical Techniques. Second ed. United States: ScienceDirect Book; 2019. pp. 384-406

[64] Baumgartner H, Falk V, Bax JJ, et al. ESC/EACTS guidelines for the management of valvular heart disease. European Heart Journal. 2017;**38**(36): 2739-2791

Section 5

Cardiac Conduction Tissue

Chapter 5

Conduction System Disorders Associated with Valvular Heart Disease and Interventions

Muhtashim Mian and Habib Rehman Khan

Abstract

The aging population of the Western world will lead to an increase in cardiac pathologies. Valvular disorders include a spectrum of progressive diseases that confers mechanical and functional impairment, including issues with the cardiac conduction system. Pacemakers are a therapeutic standard to reinstate the synchrony of cardiac contraction. Permanent pacemakers are often required for severe, chronic presentations and have been effective in nullifying symptoms and improving cardiac function. Yet, these devices impart new risks and complications that require additional interventions. However, recent advancements in leadless pacemakers and cardiac resynchronization therapy provide a novel approach to applying pacemaker technology and have been shown to reduce associated risks and improve patient outcomes.

Keywords: aortic stenosis (AS), mitral regurgitation (MR), infectious endocarditis (IE), mitral valve, aortic valve, left ventricular hypertrophy

1. Introduction

Amongst all cardiac procedures carried out in the United States, it is estimated that 10–20% were related to Valvular Heart Disease (VHD) [1]. Moreover, given the increasing age of the Western and developed population, the burden of VHD is expected to increase. As VHDs become severe and/or symptomatic, surgery is eventually required. There are invasive and minimally invasive percutaneous interventions for valve repair and surgery, with varying conductive tissue complications. Conversely, treatment for the underlying conductive disease (i.e. pacemakers) has valvular complications. This review will outline these complications.

2. Conduction tissue anatomy

The heart's pumping action is mediated by specialized muscle fibers known as cardiomyocytes. Unlike typical myocytes, they possess the capacity to self-initiate an electrical impulse for muscular contraction. They are regulated by a highly specialized group of cells compacted to form the conduction system (**Figure 1**).

The sinoatrial (SA) node (the pacemaker) is the site of impulse generation and is located between the superior vena cava (SVC) and the right atrium (RA).

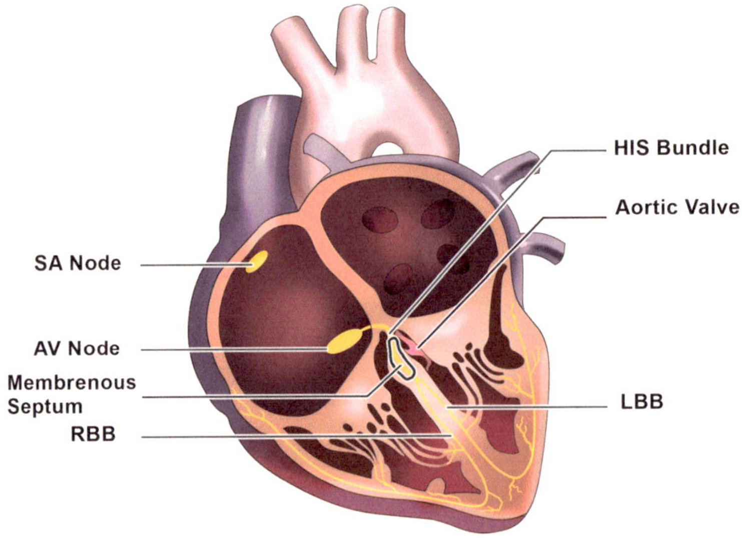

Figure 1.
Normal conduction system of the heart.

The generated electrical pulse propagates from the SA node and travels along the myocardium of the left and right atria, stimulating contraction and propelling blood from the atria into the ventricles. The electrical signal then travels along specialized cardiac muscle fibers to the atrioventricular (AV) node. The specialized cells that guide the signal are collectively known as the internodal pathways; 3 of which originate from the RA and 1 from the left atrium (LA). Upon reaching the AV node (AVN), the electrical impulse slows down, allowing the adequate filling of the ventricles before contraction. The electrical impulse then travels to a group of specialized cardiac cells called the His Bundle, which divides along the septum into left and right branches terminating into the Purkinje fibers. Signal transduction along these fibers results in ventricular contraction to expel the blood from the heart and into pulmonary (from the right ventricle) and systemic (from the left ventricle) circulation.

3. Conduction tissue disease

Cardiac conduction tissue disorders are a group of disorders that impair the above system. They are classified according to the area affected by disease processes as shown in **Figure 2**.

3.1 Sinus node dysfunction

Sinus Node Dysfunction (SND) refers to the ailment in the SA node's ability to generate electrical impulses. SND primarily affects older individuals (over 65 years of age), however, individuals of any age can present with it. As such, the most common pathological mechanism is degenerative fibrosis of the SA node and its subsequent remodeling. Any factors that affect the ionic currents of the pacemaker cells can lead to the presentation of SND. These include beta-blockers, calcium channel blockers and antiarrhythmic medication. SND is often associated with electrolyte imbalances such as hyperkalemia, hypokalemia or hypercalcemia.

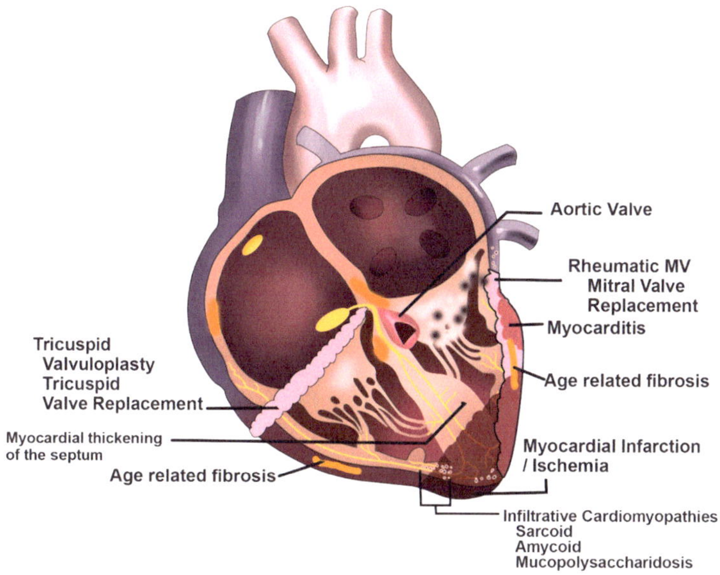

Figure 2.
Conditions associated with conduction system abnormalities.

A characteristic form of SND is a tachycardia-bradycardia syndrome, whereby tachycardia persists but devolves into severe bradycardia either spontaneously or as an attempt to medically manage tachycardia [2]. SND can also present with varying degrees of severity with differing ECG findings. First-degree SA block is asymptomatic and cannot be detected on the ECG. The second-degree SA block is characterized by a dropped P wave but is not associated with any change in the P–P interval. Third-degree SA block is complete dysfunction of the SA pacemaker cells with no discernable P wave on the ECG (23).

3.2 Atrioventricular block

Atrioventricular block (AVB) refers to disorders whereby the propagation of impulse generated in the SA node is impaired from propagating to the ventricles in varying degrees. AVB can be secondary to defined cardiomyopathy but often is idiopathic. AVB can also be a consequence of intervention for valvular disease. Diagnosis and progression of AVB are determined by the abnormalities in the AV electrical activity and which cardiac structure is affected.

First-degree AVB (AVB I) is associated with a prolonged PR interval, indicating a delay in the AVN, which is typically considered benign due to normal ventricular filling. However, the patient may become symptomatic with increased activity due to deterioration of AVN conduction associated with a faster heart rate. Moreover, cases with marked first-degree AVB (delay greater than 300 ms) can result in shorter diastolic time and produce "pacemaker-like syndrome" symptoms. This is a major mechanism of increased risk of future atrial fibrillation and indicates the need for pacemaker implantation [3].

Second-degree AVB (AVB II) is further sub-classed into Mobitz Type I (Wenckebach) and Mobitz Type II. Mobitz Type I AVB classically presents with progressive prolongation of the PR intervals until there is a non-conducted P wave. Mobitz Type I AVB typically affects the AV node itself and is deemed to be benign and reversible. Mobitz Type II presents with constant PR intervals that are preceded and followed by a non-conducted P wave. Mobitz Type II AVB is a challenging diagnosis as the PR interval may appear normal and the mere presence of non-conducted P waves is not an automatic indication of Type II AVB. Type II AVB affects the conduction system distal to the AV node in the His Bundle system.

Third-degree AVB (AVB III) is also known as complete AVB in which there is complete dissociation between atrial and ventricular conductive tissue. Thus, any presence of QRS complexes is independent of the generation of P waves. Ventricular contraction is due to intrinsic junctional or ventricular rhythm and poses the greatest risk of hemodynamic instability and fatal cardiac arrhythmias resulting in death.

3.3 Left bundle branch block

Left bundle branch block (LBBB) refers to impaired conduction of branches of the His Bundle system, specifically the narrow anterior fascicle and the broader posterior fascicle. Typically, LBBB presents with prolonged QRS (>120 ms), absent Q wave in V_6 and rS complexes in V_1-V_2 [4]. In isolation, LBBBs are asymptomatic and confer no risk to the patient. However, LBBBs underlying etiology is dilated cardiomyopathy, which itself can be caused by ischemic, infective, infiltrative or valvular cardiac disease [5]. Moreover, it has been shown that individuals with LBBB and incomplete AVB carry a greater risk of progressing to complete AVB [5].

Whilst there is no complete treatment for LBBB, cardiac resynchronization therapy (Section 5.3) has been shown to benefit patients who present with heart failure alongside LBBB (27).

4. Conductive tissue disorders associated with Valvular interventions

Historically, heart surgery has been the only option amongst patients with symptomatic severe valvular heart disease. However, for patients that are not surgical candidates, minimally invasive transcatheter approaches are increasingly employed for valve repair and/or replacement. Each of these interventions can be associated with differing rates of Conductive System Disorders (CSDs). Complete or high-degree AVB is a particular concern, for which guidelines from the American College of Cardiology/American Heart Association recommend permanent pacemakers if there is no resolution after 1-week post-surgical intervention [6]. The conductive tissue complications following invasive and minimally-invasive VHD interventions will be outlined here.

4.1 Aortic valve interventions

Transcatheter aortic valve replacement (TAVR) is a minimally invasive technique for symptomatic severe AS that has gained wide adoption, having been performed in over 400,000 patients worldwide as of 2017 [7]. While initially reserved for patients at high surgical risk, TAVR has shown non-inferior or superiority to SAVR for all-cause mortality, cardiovascular mortality and stroke amongst medium and low surgical risk populations up to 5-year follow-up [8, 9]. However, TAVR has lower valve durability and higher rates of paravalvular leaks and CSD, namely left bundle branch blocks and AVBs requiring pacemaker insertion [8–10]. The rates of pacemaker insertion post-TAVR vary based on type (self-expanding vs. balloon expanding) and generation of valve used. Meta-analyses have reported pacemaker insertion rates of approximately 3.8–6.5% for balloon-expanding vs. 12–25.8% for self-expanding valves [11, 12]. The self-expanding valves do have increased effective orifice area at the cost of worse rates of CSD, though the clinical significance of better orifice area is not born out in short to medium-term studies done thus far [11]. The mechanism of conductive tissue disruption is thought to be from injury to the AV node while the deployment of the valve into the left ventricular outflow tract; self-expanding valves by their nature exert a greater radial and compressive force on peri-valvular conductive tissue over time which is likely results in the observed outcome of increased pacemaker requirement. There is ongoing research about the predictors of pacemaker requirement following TAVR in either type of valve, but strong associations include male sex, baseline Mobitz type 1, baseline wide QRS, depth of valve implant, and intraprocedural AV block [13–15]. Given the increased risk of LBBB post-TAVR, pre-existing right bundle disease (RBBB or bifascicular block) predisposes to complete AVB requiring pacemaker [13].

Surgical Aortic Valve Replacement (SAVR) is a well-established procedure for the treatment of severe aortic stenosis or regurgitation. An important benefit of SAVR over TAVR is valve durability, particularly with mechanical valves as these are not possible currently with TAVR. SAVR has traditionally been performed using sutured valves, with post-surgical pacemaker requirement in 2–4% of cases [16–18]. However, with the advent of TAVR, sutureless valves (similar in concept to balloon-expanded TAVR valves) are increasingly being used in SAVR as they minimize procedure and hospital time [19]. Given the stent-expanding nature of sutureless SAVR, they result in higher rates of pacemaker requirement compared to conventional SAVR [20, 21]. There are limited trials comparing SAVR to TAVR; many have shown worse rates of pacemaker requirement in TAVR but the TAVR cohorts include both self-expanding and balloon-expanded valves [22–24]. When comparing balloon-expanded TAVR to sutureless SAVR however, the rates of pacemaker requirement were similar over a two-year follow-up [25]. More studies are quired for recommendations between sutureless SAVR and TAVR.

4.2 Mitral valve interventions

The Mitral valve (MV) is significantly more complex than the aortic valve due to the papillary muscles and chordae tendinea that tether leaflets to the left ventricle, as well as its ovoid annulus. The definitive treatment for severe MV stenosis or regurgitation is surgical replacement or repair, but this is limited by surgical risk. The incidence of AVBs following Mitral valve surgical replacement is up to 18% AVB I, 5% AVB II, and 5% AVB III [26–29]. Following mitral valve surgical replacement, a permanent pacemaker is required in approximately 2–11% of cases [30]. Notably, Mitral valve surgical replacement is associated with an approximately 20% higher risk of CSD requiring a permanent pacemaker compared to aortic valve surgical replacement [28]. This is likely related to the proximity of the mitral valve (MV) annulus to the AV node, Specifically, the posterolateral artery which supplies the AV node is adjacent to the mitral annulus and may be damaged intra or post-surgically.

While AVBs are well-document in the surgical intervention of MV, Conductive tissue abnormalities are uncommon following mitral transcatheter edge-to-edge repair (TEER). A case report of a patient with a baseline trifascicular block did show complete AVB following the MitraClip procedure with a proposed mechanism of injury being the instrumentation of MV apparatus during the procedure [31]. Similarly, a case reported the development of Mobitz type II following the Cardioband procedure subsequently degrading into complete AVB. The mechanism of conductive tissue injury was thought to be the deployment of screws into the MV annulus to anchor the Cardioband system. These case reports highlight the significance of MV annulus instrumentation. Nevertheless, transcatheter mitral valve repair is generally not complicated by CSDs.

Transcatheter Mitral Valve Replacement (TMVR) is technically challenging given the complexity of the mitral valve apparatus. Given its infancy, several TMVR systems are undergoing development and research and as of 2020, ACC/AHA guidelines for VHD do not offer any recommendations for TMVR [10]. The TMVR techniques currently in development vary in the approach to valve deployment (transapical vs. transfemoral/transeptal) and mechanism of expansion into valve apparatus (self-expanding vs. balloon-expanding), which theoretically could have implications for CSDs. Yet, AV blocks or bundle branch blocks have not been reported as complications post-valve deployment short-term in feasibility studies thus far [32–35].

4.3 Tricuspid valve interventions

Moderate to severe tricuspid regurgitation is often overlooked as a contributor to mortality, despite its association with increased mortality even after adjusting for LV dysfunction and pulmonary hypertension [36]. It can be categorized as primary (congenital or acquired abnormality of tricuspid apparatus itself) or secondary (abnormality of tricuspid apparatus occurring as a consequence of pulmonary hypertension, right or left ventricular dysfunction). RV damage because of TR can become irreversible, suggesting the benefits of earlier intervention [37]. Surgical intervention is indicated for symptomatic patients with severe primary TR, or in asymptomatic patients with worsening RV dysfunction. Similarly, ESC guidelines recommend early consideration of surgical intervention in patients with symptomatic TR or mildly symptomatic severe TR with RV dilation [38]. However, surgical correction has significant surgery-related morbidity and mortality. Transcatheter Tricuspid Valve Interventions (TTVI) aimed at poor surgical candidates are undoing research and development and include direct annuloplasty, leaflet approximation or valve replacement. TTVIs have shown improvement in RV performance and hemodynamics up to 6 months post-procedure, as well as improvement in HF rehospitalizations and survival up to 1-year post-procedure. An expected complication of TTVIs is heart block, though this has not been a widely report complication in preliminary reports [39, 40]. As the TTVI experience improves, it may become an effective strategy to treat pacemaker-induced TR (Section 5.5).

5. Treatment of conductive tissue disorders

Cardiac CSDs are a major cause of morbidity and mortality. Approximately 1% of the general population has CSDs necessitating permanent pacemakers (PPM), with incident rates continuing to rise each year [41]. The first implantable pacemaker by Senning in Stockholm in 1957, was an extravascular pulse generator with leads implanted into the ventricular myocardium of a patient with complete heart block. Since then, several innovations have made pacemakers more robust. Most modern pacemakers comprise a pulse generator implanted subcutaneously, that is connected to lead(s) that traverse transvenously into the myocardium of the heart chamber(s). Pacing has gained complexity and now includes dual chamber pacing (right atrium and ventricle), continuous resynchronization therapy (CRT), leadless pacing and most recently, conductive tissue pacing as shown in **Figure 3**.

5.1 Single and dual chamber pacemakers

Single chamber pacemakers are the simplest form of pacing: they have a single lead implanted into the myocardium of the right atrium or the right ventricle

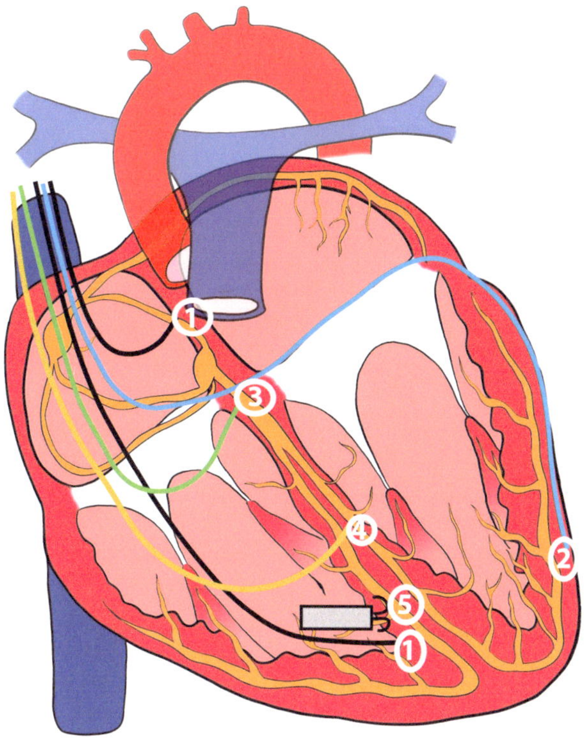

Figure 3.
Treatment of conduction system disease with different types of pacing techniques.

(**Figure 4A**). Single lead pacing is a cure for symptomatic conductive tissue disorders in the short term. However, it was not physiologic as a ventricular contraction occurred irrespective of atrial activity; with loss of synchronized atrial contraction in ventricular single chamber pacing, the ventricular filling would theoretically be diminished. Thus, Ventricular single chamber pacemakers are now primarily used in patients with poor atrial ejection fraction, namely persistent atrial fibrillation, where the atrial mechanical coupling is compromised. Atrial single-lead pacemakers are theoretically also useful in treating isolated sinus node dysfunction but are rarely used as there is usually concomitant AV and sub-AV node disease.

To preserve atrial and ventricular synchrony, dual-chamber pacemakers were developed, whereby both an atrial and ventricular lead are implanted into the myocardium (**Figure 4B**). Improved synchrony by dual-chamber pacemakers translates to improved outcomes in some but not all populations. A 2004 Cochrane review of 26 studies comparing dual to single-chamber pacemakers revealed a significant reduction in atrial fibrillation and a non-significant reduction in heart failure, stroke and mortality with dual-chamber pacing [42]. Interestingly, amongst elderly patients, there was no difference in clinical outcomes between single and dual chamber pacemakers, likely reflecting higher rates of baseline atrial fibrillation in this age group [43].

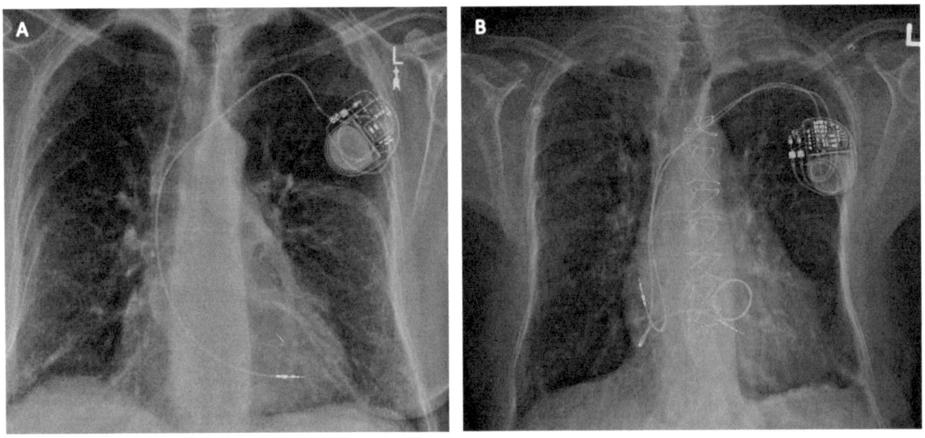

Figure 4.
(A) CXR showing a single chamber pacemaker with pacing lead placed in the RV. (B). CXR showing a dual chamber pacemaker following mitral valve replacement and tricuspid valve annuloplasty.

5.2 Leadless pacemaker

Leadless pacing is a novel therapy whereby an electrical impulse generator is percutaneously implanted directly into the myocardium, obviating the need for leads (**Figure 5**). The lack of leads and subcutaneous pulse generator has the theoretical benefit of avoiding lead-related (ex. lead infections, lead failure, tricuspid regurgitation) and subcutaneous pocket (ex. Pocket infections, hematoma) complications.

At this time, the majority of literature is on two leadless pacemakers: Nanostim (St. Jude Medical, St. Paul, MN,USA) and Micra (Medtronic, Minneapolis, MN). Nanostim had promising results from initial trials but was recalled due to premature battery failure and spontaneous detachment from the myocardium. For these reasons, it did not gain FDA approval and is not currently being implanted. An updated Nansostim system called Aveir VR gained FDA approval in March 2022 but no trials have been completed thus far. As Micra is the only FDA-approved leadless pacemaker with short to medium-term data, it will be the focus of this review. Although there are no clinical trials directly comparing Micra to transvenous

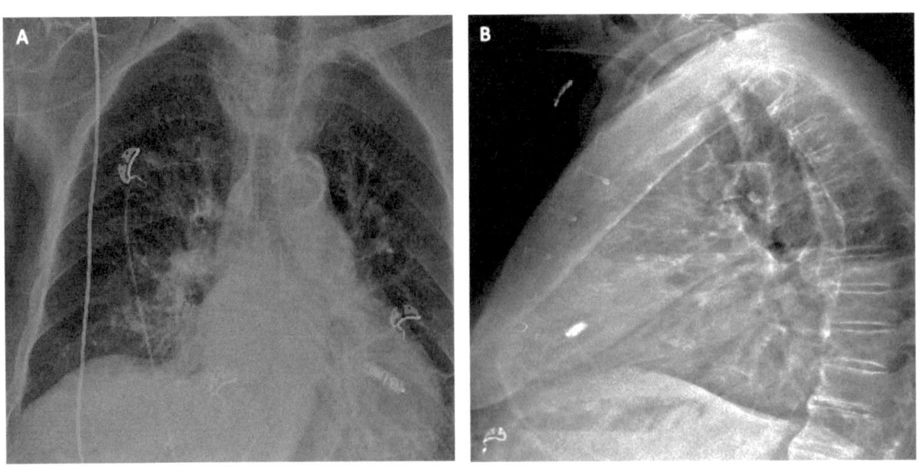

Figure 5.
CXR of a leadless pacemaker. An anteroposterior (A) and a lateral (B) view show the position of the leadless pacemaker.

pacing, observational studies up to 1-year post-implant have shown a significant reduction in the odds of developing infectious complications compared to transvenous pacing, while maintaining electrophysiologic pacing parameters [44–46]. Leadless pacing shows promise in reducing complications, but long-term trials are needed to verify electrophysiologic stability.

5.3 Cardiac resynchronization therapy

CRT is a pacing strategy to improve dyssynchronous left and right ventricular contraction; it involves biventricular pacing (RV and LV lead as shown in **Figure 6**) and can also be achieved in left-sided persistent SVC, congenital heart disease and anomalous coronary sinus veins [47–49]. Cardiac mechanical desynchrony is of particular concern amongst select patients with heart failure with reduced ejection fraction (HFrEF) [50]. Patients with HFrEF undergo cardiac remodeling over time which results in electrical dysregulation and interventricular delays ultimately causing dyssynchronous contraction of the right and left ventricles and poor cardiac function; these interventricular delays can be in the form of left bundle branch block or non-specific electrical conduction delays that increased QRS duration. Indeed, QRS duration correlates with worsening heart failure and sudden cardiac death and death from any cause [50]. CRT is an effective strategy to mitigate interventricular delays as the electrical generator can be programmed to initiate optimal timing of contraction for each ventricle. CRT has been shown to reduce mortality by up to 36% compared to medical therapy alone in patients with interventricular delay [51]. Given the evidence, ACCF/AHA/HRS guidelines suggest CRT for patients with Left Ventricular Ejection Fraction <35%, sinus rhythm, LBBB with QRS > 150 ms and NYHA class 2–4 symptoms on goal-directed medical therapy (class 1) [52].

Amongst HFrEF patients who would otherwise benefit from CRT, the presence of atrial fibrillation (AF) can be problematic. The rapid ventricular response or irregularity of AF can interfere with biventricular pacing capture rendering CRT ineffective in up to 67% of patients with persistent AF [53]. One solution to this dilemma is ablation followed by biventricular pacing. A recent meta-analysis showed worse mortality in AF patients compared to normal sinus patients that underwent CRT [54]. However, when AF patients underwent ablation, all-cause mortality

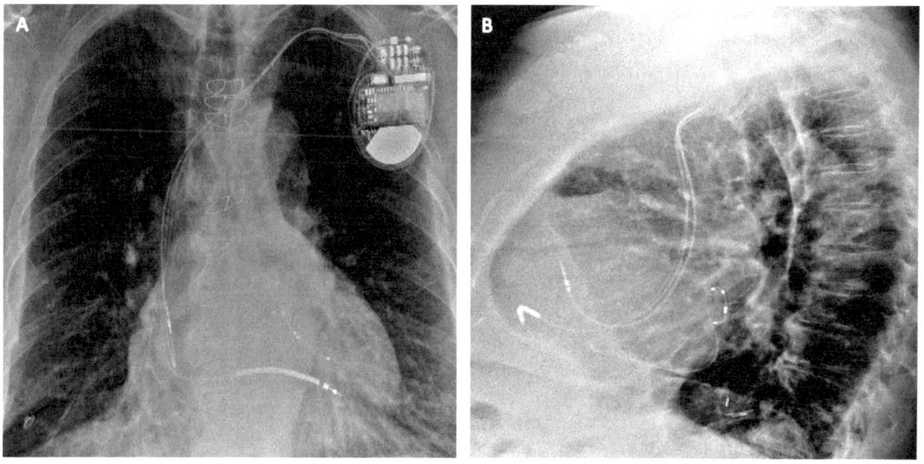

Figure 6.
CXR of CRT. An anteroposterior and lateral view showing the leads in the right atrium, right ventricle and a quadripolar left ventricular pacing lead through the coronary sinus.

was not different between the normal sinus and AF patients undergoing CRT [54]. Most recent ACCF/AHA/HRS guidelines recommend CRT for AF patients that a) otherwise meet CRT criteria as above and b) AV nodal ablation or pharmacologic rate control will achieve near 100% ventricular pacing with CRT (class IIa) [52].

5.4 Conductive system pacing

International guidelines for pacing currently recommend the above conventional myocardial pacing whereby slow-conducting myocytes are activated and therefore only indirectly activate the fast-conductive cardiac tissue (i.e. His-Purkinje network). Direct conduction system pacing (CSP) is emerging as an alternative approach to myocardial pacing; by directly activating conductive tissue, CSP has the theoretical benefit of mitigating electrical and mechanical ventricular desynchrony.

Two methods of CSP that have garnered attention are His Bundle Pacing (HBP) whereby a lead is inserted proximally close to His bundle, and Left Bundle Branch area Pacing (LBBaP) whereby a lead is inserted more distally close to the LBB (**Figure 7**). Wang et al. recently showed that HBP was feasible and safe with improvements in LVEF in patients with persistent AF and HFrEF who indicated implantable cardioverter defibrillator [55]. Abdelrahman et al. showed that patients with HBP had better survival and heart failure hospitalization rates compared to conventional RV pacing [56]. While HBP can be effective, it can be technically challenging given the small target area for lead placement, with longer procedure times even amongst experienced electrophysiologists compared to conventional pacing [57]. Furthermore, HBP has higher rates of lead dislodgement, up to twice as compared to conventional RV pacing [58]. LBBaP may be a better alternative in some patient populations. For instance, in patients requiring AV node ablation LBBaP is technically less challenging and pacing output to correct the left bundle branch block is lower. However, given the relative recency of CSP, there is currently a paucity of data including complications, such that international cardiology societies have yet to make recommendations [59].

One possible advantage of CSP over conventional pacing is the concept of synchrony. While right ventricular pacing is effective for the treatment of bradycardia and syncope, this approach can lead to electrical and mechanical desynchrony (particularly between ventricles) with the remodeling of the heart long-term; the broad consequences are higher rates of atrial fibrillation, heart failure and mortality [60, 61]. As previously described, Cardiac Resynchronization therapy (CRT) can mitigate hemodynamic and structural complications associated with only right ventricular pacing. Clinical trials have demonstrated that CRT reverses remodeling, and improves left ventricular ejection fraction (LVEF) and overall mortality in patients with reduced ejection fraction heart failure (HFrEF) [62, 63]. However, up to 40% of patients eligible for CRT demonstrate "non-response" (i.e. poor improvement in NYHA class, QRS duration, or echocardiographic parameters) [64]. Furthermore, while conventional CRT does improve QRS duration, it does not return it to a range seen in patients with intact conduction tissue, suggesting better therapeutic benefits with shorter QRS [65]. Whether CSP can be used as an alternative to, or as rescue therapy for patients with an indication for CRT remains to be seen. Several centers, including our own, are undergoing trials to address this question.

5.5 Tricuspid regurgitation following pacing

As mentioned in Section 4.3, TR is an independent cause of mortality [66]. Pacemaker-associated TR can be primary TR by direct damage of the tricuspid valve by leads, secondary TR by RV dilation and dysfunction due to pacemaker

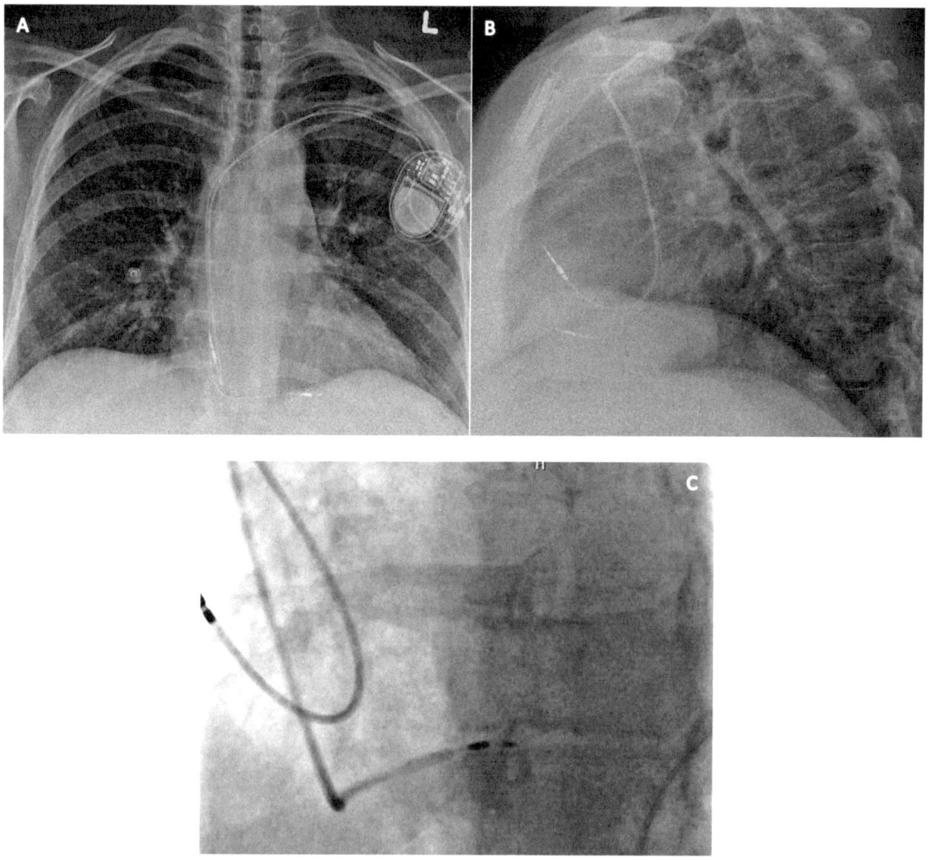

Figure 7.
CXR of dual chamber pacemaker. An anteroposterior and lateral view showing the position of a dual chamber pacemaker. RV lead is placed in the apical position (A) in comparison to placement at the region of LBBAP (B). Contrast injection through the delivery sheath showing the lead penetrating the RV septum to successfully deliver LBBAP.

cardiomyopathy, or a combination of both. As TR is a major complication of pacing, prevention of TR is an important consideration.

Leadless pacemakers (see 5.2) have the theoretical benefit of minimizing primary damage to the tricuspid valve. However, Beurskens et al. showed that 12-month follow-up for leadless pacing had comparable rates of TR to the dual-chamber paced group, suggesting that lead-related damage to the tricuspid valve may not be the primary mechanism of TR following pacing [67]. The TR observed in leadless pacing may be due to RV dysfunction from pacemaker cardiomyopathy or damage to the tricuspid apparatus while crossing the tricuspid valve during implantation [68]. One way to avoid tricuspid apparatus entirely is to implant lead into the left ventricle via the coronary sinus. Schliefer et al. tested this hypothesis in a prospective trial comparing rates of TR at 12 months between pacing at RV-apex vs. RV-septum vs. LV-coronary sinus; coronary sinus pacing failed to achieve a statistically significant reduction of TR [69]. More studies over longer follow-ups are required to verify these findings.

6. Conclusion

Given the aging population of the Western world, the burden of Valvular Heart Diseases is predicted to increase. Advancement and development of new percutaneous valvular interventions have been a boon for patients, particularly those deemed to be poor surgical candidates. Alongside these percutaneous valvular interventions are increased rates of CSDs, often requiring artificial pacing. Pacing techniques have also seen rapid advancements, with the advent of CRT, leadless pacing and conductive tissue pacing. Each of these has merit and warrants further research, particularly in the need to tailor different pacing modalities to different valvular interventions.

Abbreviations

AF	Atrial Fibrillation
AVN	Atrioventricular Node
AVB	Atrioventricular Block
CRT	cardiac resynchronization therapy
CSD	conduction system disorder
CSP	conduction system pacing
HBP	His Bundle Pacing
HFrEF	heart failure with reduced ejection fraction
LA	Left Atrium
LBBaP	Left Bundle Branch area Pacing
LBBB	Left Bundle Branch Block
LVEF	left ventricular ejection fraction
MV	Mitral valve
NYHA	New York Heart Association
RA	Right Atrium
RBBB	Right Bundle Branch Block
SA	Sinoatrial Node
SAVR	Surgical Aortic Valve Replacement
SND	Sinus Node Dysfunction
SVC	Superior Vena Cava
TAVR	Transcatheter aortic valve replacement
TEER	transcatheter edge-to-edge repair
TMVR	Transcatheter Mitral Valve Replacement
TR	Tricuspid Regurgitation
TTVI	Transcatheter Tricuspid Valve Interventions
VHD	Valvular Heart Disease

Author details

Muhtashim Mian and Habib Rehman Khan*
London Health Sciences Centre, London, Canada
Schulich School of Medicine and Dentistry, University of Western Ontario

*Address all correspondence to: habib.khan@lhsc.on.ca

References

[1] Iung B, Vahanian A. Epidemiology of valvular heart disease in the adult. Nature Reviews. Cardiology. 2011;**8**:162-172

[2] Sick Sinus Syndrome: A Review. Available from: https://www.aafp.org/pubs/afp/issues/2013/0515/p691.html. [Accessed: July 17, 2022]

[3] Cheng S, Keyes MJ, Larson MG, McCabe EL, Newton-Cheh C, Levy D, et al. Long-term outcomes in individuals with prolonged PR interval or first-degree atrioventricular block. JAMA. 2009;**301**:2571-2577

[4] Nikoo MH, Aslani A, Jorat MV. LBBB: State-of-the-art criteria. International Cardiovascular Research Journal. 2013;**7**:39

[5] Francia P, Balla C, Paneni F, Volpe M. Left bundle-branch block—Pathophysiology, prognosis, and clinical management. Clinical Cardiology. 2007;**30**:110-115

[6] Gregoratos G, Abrams J, Epstein AE, Freedman RA, Hayes DL, Hlatky MA, et al. ACC/AHA/NASPE 2002 guideline update for implantation of cardiac pacemakers and Antiarrhythmia devices: Summary article. A report of the American College of Cardiology/American Heart Association task force on practice guidelines (ACC/AHA/NASPE committee to update the 1998 pacemaker guidelines). Circulation. 2002;**106**:2145-2161

[7] Kourkoveli P, Spargias K, Hahalis G. Perspective open access • TAVR in 2017-what we know? What to expect? Journal of Geriatric Cardiology. 2018;**15**:55-60

[8] Kolte D, Vlahakes GJ, Palacios IF, Sakhuja R, Passeri JJ, Inglessis I, et al. Transcatheter versus surgical aortic valve replacement in low-risk patients. Journal of the American College of Cardiology. 2019;**74**:1532-1540

[9] Siontis GCM, Overtchouk P, Cahill TJ, Modine T, Prendergast B, Praz F, et al. Transcatheter aortic valve implantation vs. surgical aortic valve replacement for treatment of symptomatic severe aortic stenosis: An updated meta-analysis. European Heart Journal. 2019;**40**:3143-3153

[10] Otto CM, Nishimura RA, Bonow RO, Carabello BA, Erwin JP, Gentile F, et al. 2020 ACC/AHA guideline for the Management of Patients with Valvular Heart Disease: A report of the American College of Cardiology/American Heart Association joint committee on clinical practice guidelines. Circulation, 2021; 143: E72–E227.

[11] Lee HA, Chou AH, Wu VCC, Chen DY, Lee HF, Lee KT, et al. Balloon-expandable versus self-expanding transcatheter aortic valve replacement for bioprosthetic dysfunction: A systematic review and meta-analysis. PLoS One. 2020;**15**:e0233894

[12] van Belle E, Vincent F, Labreuche J, Auffret V, Debry N, Lefèvre T, et al. Balloon-expandable versus self-expanding Transcatheter aortic valve replacement. Circulation. 2020;**141**:243-259

[13] Ullah W, Zahid S, Zaidi SR, Sarvepalli D, Haq S, Roomi S, et al. Predictors of permanent pacemaker implantation in patients undergoing Transcatheter aortic valve replacement - a systematic review and meta-analysis. Journal of the American Heart Association. 2021;**10**:20906

[14] Nazif TM, Dizon JM, Hahn RT, Xu K, Babaliaros V, Douglas PS, et al. Predictors and clinical outcomes of permanent pacemaker implantation

after transcatheter aortic valve replacement: The PARTNER (placement of AoRtic TraNscathetER valves) trial and registry. JACC. Cardiovascular Interventions. 2015;**8**:60-69

[15] Kiani S, Kamioka N, Black GB, Lu MLR, Lisko JC, Rao B, et al. Development of a risk score to predict new pacemaker implantation after Transcatheter aortic valve replacement. JACC. Cardiovascular Interventions. 2019;**12**:2133-2142

[16] Limongelli G, Ducceschi V, D'Andrea A, Renzulli A, Sarubbi B, de Feo M, et al. Risk factors for pacemaker implantation following aortic valve replacement: A single Centre experience. Heart. 2003;**89**:901-904

[17] Bagur R, Manazzoni JM, Dumont É, Doyle D, Perron J, Dagenais F, et al. Permanent pacemaker implantation following isolated aortic valve replacement in a large cohort of elderly patients with severe aortic stenosis. Heart. 2011;**97**:1687-1694

[18] van Mieghem NM, Head SJ, de Jong W, van Domburg RT, Serruys PW, de Jaegere PP, et al. Persistent annual permanent pacemaker implantation rate after surgical aortic valve replacement in patients with severe aortic stenosis. The Annals of Thoracic Surgery. 2012;**94**:1143-1149

[19] Meco M, Montisci A, Miceli A, Panisi P, Donatelli F, Cirri S, et al. Sutureless perceval aortic valve versus conventional stented bioprostheses: Meta-analysis of postoperative and midterm results in isolated aortic valve replacement. Journal of the American Heart Association. 2018;**7**:e006091. DOI: 10.1161/JAHA.117.006091

[20] Hurley ET, O'Sullivan KE, Segurado R, Hurley JP. A meta-analysis examining differences in short-term outcomes between Sutureless and conventional aortic valve prostheses. Innovations (Phila). 2015;**10**:375-382

[21] Phan K, Tsai Y-C, Niranjan N, Bouchard D, Carrel TP, Dapunt OE, et al. Sutureless aortic valve replacement: A systematic review and meta-analysis. Annals of Cardiothoracic Surgery. 2015;**4**:e46

[22] Muneretto C, Solinas M, Folliguet T, di Bartolomeo R, Repossini A, Laborde F, et al. Sutureless versus transcatheter aortic valves in elderly patients with aortic stenosis at intermediate risk: A multi-institutional study. The Journal of Thoracic and Cardiovascular Surgery. 2022;**163**:925-935.e5

[23] Muneretto C, Alfieri O, Cesana BM, Bisleri G, de Bonis M, di Bartolomeo R, et al. A comparison of conventional surgery, transcatheter aortic valve replacement, and sutureless valves in "real-world" patients with aortic stenosis and intermediate- to high-risk profile. The Journal of Thoracic and Cardiovascular Surgery. 2015;**150**:1570-1579

[24] Abdel-Wahab M, Fujita B, Frerker C, Bauer T, Beckmann A, Bekeredjian R, et al. Transcatheter versus rapid-deployment aortic valve replacement: A propensity-matched analysis from the German aortic valve registry. Cardiovascular Interventions. 2020;**13**:2642-2654

[25] Leon MB, Mack MJ, Hahn RT, Thourani VH, Makkar R, Kodali SK, et al. Outcomes 2 years after Transcatheter aortic valve replacement in patients at low surgical risk. Journal of the American College of Cardiology. 2021;**77**:1149-1161

[26] Berdajs D, Schurr UP, Wagner A, Seifert B, Turina MI, Genoni M. Incidence and pathophysiology of atrioventricular block following mitral valve replacement and ring annuloplasty. European Journal of Cardio-Thoracic Surgery. 2008;**34**(1): 55-61. DOI: 10.1016/j.ejcts.2008.03.051

[27] Meimoun P, Zeghdi R, D'Attelis N, Berrebi A, Braunberger E, Deloche A, et al. Frequency, predictors, and consequences of atrioventricular block after mitral valve repair. The American Journal of Cardiology. 2002;**89**:1062-1066

[28] Leyva F, Qiu T, Mcnulty D, Evison F, Marshall H, Gasparini M. Long-term requirement for pacemaker implantation after cardiac valve replacement surgery. Heart Rhythm. 2017;**14, 4**:529-534. DOI: 10.1016/j.hrthm.2016.11.029

[29] Merin O, Ilan M, Oren A, Fink D, Deeb M, Bitran D, et al. Permanent pacemaker implantation following cardiac surgery: Indications and long-term follow-up. Pacing and Clinical Electrophysiology. 2009;**32**:7-12

[30] Ghauri H, Iqbal R, Ahmed S, Ashraf A, Khan MSQ, Malik J, et al. Predictors of permanent pacemaker insertion after mitral valve replacement: A systematic review. PACE - Pacing and Clinical Electrophysiology. 2022;**45**:681-687

[31] Erinne I, Theertham AK, Maleki K, Chen C, Russo M, Hakeem A. Complete atrioventricular block: A rare complication of MitraClip implantation. JACC Case Reports. 2021;**3**:772-777

[32] Alkhouli M, Alqahtani F, Aljohani S. Transcatheter mitral valve replacement: An evolution of a revolution. Journal of Thoracic Disease. 2017;**9**:S668-S672

[33] Bapat V, Rajagopal V, Meduri C, Farivar RS, Walton A, Duffy SJ, et al. Early experience with new Transcatheter mitral valve replacement. Journal of the American College of Cardiology. 2018;**71**:12-21

[34] Webb JG, Murdoch DJ, Boone RH, Moss R, Attinger-Toller A, Blanke P, et al. Percutaneous Transcatheter mitral valve replacement: First-in-human experience with a new Transseptal system. Journal of the American College of Cardiology. 2019;**73**:1239-1246

[35] Makkar R, O'Neill W, Whisenant B, Guerrero M, Feldman T, Rihal C, et al. TCT-8 updated 30-day outcomes for the U.S. early feasibility study of the SAPIEN M3 transcatheter mitral valve replacement system. Journal of the American College of Cardiology. 2019;**74**:B8

[36] Nath J, Foster E, Heidenreich PA. Impact of tricuspid regurgitation on long-term survival. Journal of the American College of Cardiology. 2004;**43**:405-409

[37] Dreyfus J, Ghalem N, Garbarz E, Cimadevilla C, Nataf P, Vahanian A, et al. Timing of referral of patients with severe isolated tricuspid valve regurgitation to surgeons (from a French Nationwide database). The American Journal of Cardiology. 2018;**122**:323-326

[38] Riesenhuber M, Spannbauer A, Gwechenberger M, Pezawas T, Schukro C, Stix G, et al. Pacemaker lead-associated tricuspid regurgitation in patients with or without pre-existing right ventricular dilatation. Clinical Research in Cardiology. 2021;**110**:884-894

[39] Hahn RT, Kodali S, Fam N, Bapat V, Bartus K, Rodés-Cabau J, et al. Early multinational experience of Transcatheter tricuspid valve replacement for treating severe tricuspid regurgitation. JACC. Cardiovascular Interventions. 2020;**13**:2482-2493

[40] Kar S, Noureddin N, Aboulhosn J, Mahmzi Y, Coluzzi A, Tobis J, et al. Rapid pacing using the guidewire during Transcatheter tricuspid valve in valve implantation. Journal of Structural Heart Disease. 2017;**3**:157-162

[41] Bradshaw PJ, Stobie P, Knuiman MW, Briffa TG, Hobbs MST. Trends in the incidence and prevalence of cardiac pacemaker insertions in an ageing population. Open Heart. 2014;**1**:e000177. DOI: 10.1136/openhrt-2014-000177

[42] Verma N, Dandamudi S, Goldberger JJ, Lip GYH, Huffman MD. Dual chamber versus single chamber ventricular pacemakers for sick sinus syndrome and atrioventricular block. Cochrane Database of Systematic Reviews. 2004;**2004**:CD003710. DOI: 10.1002/14651858.CD003710.PUB2

[43] Toff WD, Camm AJ, Douglas J, Skehan MB. Single-chamber versus dual-chamber pacing for high-grade atrioventricular block. The New England Journal of Medicine. 2005;**353**:145-155. DOI: 101056/NEJMoa042283

[44] Vaidya VR, Dai M, Asirvatham SJ, Rea RF, Thome TM, Srivathsan K, et al. Real-world experience with leadless cardiac pacing. Pacing and Clinical Electrophysiology. 2019;**42**:366-373

[45] Ngo L, Nour D, Denman RA, Walters TE, Haqqani HM, Woodman RJ, et al. Safety and efficacy of leadless pacemakers: A systematic review and meta-analysis. Journal of the American Heart Association. 2021;**10**:19212

[46] Duray GZ, Ritter P, El-Chami M, Narasimhan C, Omar R, Tolosana JM, et al. Long-term performance of a transcatheter pacing system: 12-month results from the Micra Transcatheter pacing study. Heart Rhythm. 2017;**14**:702-709

[47] McIntosh RA, Ansari MI, Moon J, Khan HR. Delivery of cardiac resynchronization therapy via the left inferior phrenic vein: A case report. European Heart Journal - Case Reports. 2019:3, ytz144. DOI: 10.1093/ehjcr/ytz144

[48] Kuo-Wei Chiang C, Ka-Bo Chan W, So A, Yee R, Khan H. Utilizing preprocedural imaging and active fixation lead in cardiac resynchronization therapy device upgrade for persistent left superior vena cava. Heart Rhythm Case Reports. 2021;**8**:50-53

[49] Kanawati J, Kanawati AJ, Rowe MK, Khan H, Chan WK, Yee R. Utility of 3-D printing for cardiac resynchronization device implantation in congenital heart disease. Heart Rhythm Case Reports. 2020;**6**:754-756

[50] Bleeker GB, Schalij MJ, Molhoek SG, Verwey HF, Holman ER, Boersma E, et al. Relationship between QRS duration and left ventricular dyssynchrony in patients with end-stage heart failure. Journal of Cardiovascular Electrophysiology. 2004;**15**:544-549

[51] Cleland JGF, Daubert J-C, Erdmann E, Freemantle N, Gras D, Kappenberger L, et al. The effect of cardiac resynchronization on morbidity and mortality in heart failure. The New England Journal of Medicine. 2009;**352**:1539-1549. DOI: 101056/NEJMoa050496

[52] Nam EFT Jr, Tracy CM, Epstein AE, Chair V, Darbar D, et al. ACCF/AHA/HRS focused update ACCF/AHA/HRS focused update of the 2008 guidelines for device-based therapy of cardiac rhythm abnormalities a report of the American College of Cardiology Foundation/American Heart Association task force on practice guidelines and the Heart Rhythm Society. Journal of the American College of Cardiology. 2012;**126**:1784-1800

[53] Ousdigian KT, Borek PP, Koehler JL, Heywood JT, Ziegler PD, Wilkoff BL. The epidemic of inadequate biventricular pacing in patients with persistent or permanent atrial fibrillation and its association with

mortality. Circulation. Arrhythmia and Electrophysiology. 2014;7:370-376

[54] Mustafa U, Atkins J, Mina G, Dawson D, Vanchiere C, Duddyala N, et al. Outcomes of cardiac resynchronisation therapy in patients with heart failure with atrial fibrillation: A systematic review and meta-analysis of observational studies. Open Heart. 2019;**6**:e000937

[55] Lin J, Dai Y, Wang H, Li Y, Chen K, Zhang S. A comparison of left bundle branch pacing with his bundle pacing in a patient with heart failure and left bundle branch block. Heart Rhythm Case Reports. 2020;**6**:293

[56] Abdelrahman M, Subzposh FA, Beer D, Durr B, Naperkowski A, Sun H, et al. Clinical outcomes of his bundle pacing compared to right ventricular pacing. Journal of the American College of Cardiology. 2018;**71**:2319-2330

[57] Lewis AJM, Foley P, Whinnett Z, Keene D, Chandrasekaran B. His bundle pacing: A new strategy for physiological ventricular activation. Journal of the American Heart Association. 2019;**8**:10972

[58] Keene D, Arnold AD, Jastrzębski M, Burri H, Zweibel S, Crespo E, et al. His bundle pacing, learning curve, procedure characteristics, safety, and feasibility: Insights from a large international observational study. Journal of Cardiovascular Electrophysiology. 2019;**30**:1984-1993

[59] Glikson M, Nielsen JC, Kronborg MB, Michowitz Y, Auricchio A, Barbash IM, et al. 2021 ESC guidelines on cardiac pacing and cardiac resynchronization therapy. European Heart Journal. 2021;**42**(35):3427-3520. DOI: 10.1093/EURHEARTJ/EHAB364

[60] Brenyo A, Goldenberg I, Barsheshet A. The downside of right ventricular apical pacing. Indian Pacing and Electrophysiology Journal. 2012;**12**:102

[61] Lamas GA, Lee KL, Sweeney MO, Silverman R, Leon A, Yee R, et al. Ventricular pacing or dual-chamber pacing for sinus-node dysfunction. The New England Journal of Medicine. 2002;**346**:1854-1862

[62] Tang ASL, Wells GA, Talajic M, Arnold MO, Sheldon R, Connolly S, et al. Cardiac-resynchronization therapy for mild-to-moderate. Heart Failure. 2010;**363**:2385-2395. DOI: 101056/NEJMoa1009540

[63] Goldenberg I, Kutyifa V, Klein HU, Cannom DS, Brown MW, Dan A, et al. Survival with cardiac-resynchronization therapy in mild heart failure. New England Journal of Medicine. 2014;**370**:1694-1701

[64] Daubert C, Behar N, Martins RP, Mabo P, Leclercq C. Avoiding non-responders to cardiac resynchronization therapy: A practical guide. European Heart Journal. 2017;**38**:1463-1472

[65] Ali N, Shin MS, Whinnett Z. The emerging role of cardiac conduction system pacing as a treatment for heart failure. Current Heart Failure Reports. 2020;**17**:288

[66] Kanawati J, Ng ACC, Khan H, Yu C, Hyun K, Abed H, et al. Long-term follow-up of mortality and heart failure hospitalisation in patients with Intracardiac device-related tricuspid regurgitation. Heart, Lung & Circulation. 2021;**30**:692-697

[67] Beurskens NEG, Tjong FVY, de Bruin-Bon RHA, Dasselaar KJ, Kuijt WJ, Wilde AAM, et al. Impact of leadless pacemaker therapy on cardiac and atrioventricular valve function through 12 months of follow-up. Circulation. Arrhythmia and Electrophysiology.

2019;**12**:e007124. DOI: 10.1161/CIRCEP.118.007124

[68] Chang JD, Manning WJ, Ebrille E, Zimetbaum PJ. Tricuspid valve dysfunction following pacemaker or cardioverter-defibrillator implantation. Journal of the American College of Cardiology. 2017;**69**:2331-2341

[69] Schleifer JW, Pislaru SV, Lin G, Powell BD, Espinosa R, Koestler C, et al. Effect of ventricular pacing lead position on tricuspid regurgitation: A randomized prospective trial. Heart Rhythm. 2018;**15**:1009-1016

Section 6

Miscellaneous Valve Surgery

Chapter 6

Role of Concomitant Valve Surgery in Orthotopic Heart Transplant

Yasuhiro Shudo

Abstract

There remains a significant shortage of donor hearts despite an ever-increasing demand. In an effort to maximize the utilization of this scarce resource, extended criteria for donor hearts with surgically correctable abnormalities should be considered. Bench valve surgery on the donor heart prior to heart transplantation is feasible, and its implementation could enable the use of previously unsalvageable hearts, thus expanding the donor organ pool. With proper donor and recipient selection, bench valve surgery will enable the expansion of the donor pool to provide high-quality donor allografts that would otherwise have been declined. This chapter reviews the current practices employed in heart transplantation, with emphasis on the surgical technique for concomitant valve surgery in the donor heart prior to transplantation.

Keywords: orthotopic heart transplant, donor valve disease, bench valve surgery

1. Introduction

Orthotopic heart transplantation is the gold standard treatment for end-stage heart failure [1]. According to the 2019 Registry of the International Society for Heart and Lung Transplantation, approximately 5000 heart transplantations were performed from July 1, 2017, to June 30, 2018 [2] (**Figure 1**). With the increasing prevalence of heart failure, it is estimated that over 25,000 patients annually can benefit from heart transplantation [3].

There are approximately 3000 candidates on the heart transplant waiting list in the United States. The mortality rate on the waiting list is approximately 15%, and the annual number of heart transplants is approximately 2500. Thus, there remains a severe shortage of donor hearts despite an ever-increasing demand. In an effort to maximize the utilization of this scarce resource, extended criteria for donor hearts with surgically correctable abnormalities should be considered [4]. Although there is consensus that mild valvular abnormalities in the donor may be amenable to repair or replacement on the bench [5], only a limited number of reports [6–16] in the literature exist, and a standardized technique has not been well established or adopted.

This chapter reviews the current practices employed in heart transplantation, with emphasis on the surgical technique for concomitant valve surgery in the donor heart prior to transplantation.

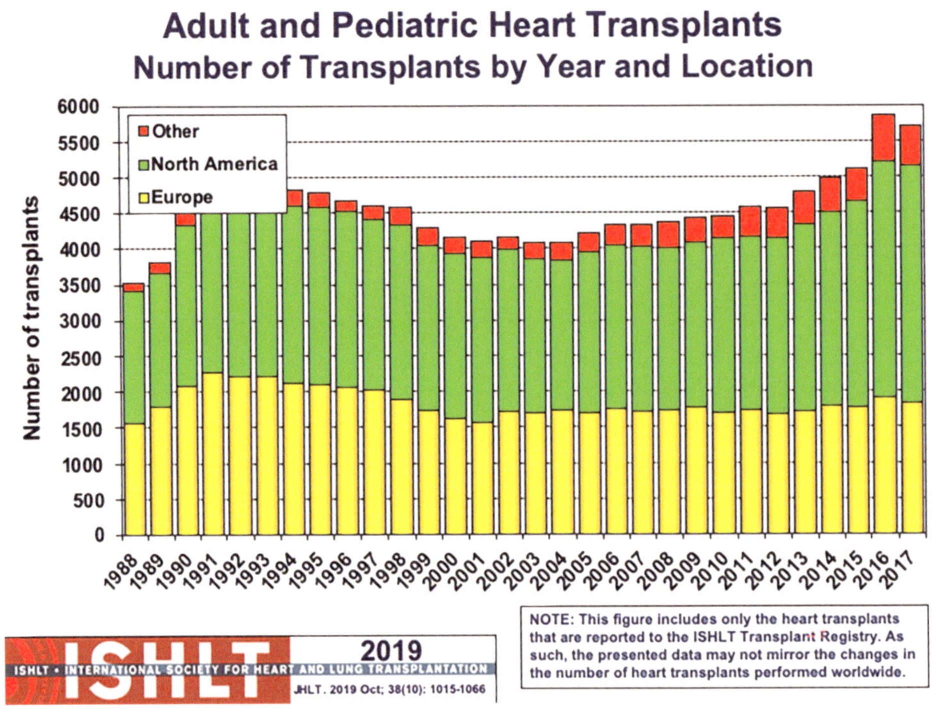

Figure 1.
Number of adult and pediatric patients who underwent orthotopic heart transplantation by year, from the International Society for Heart and Lung Transplantation 2019 report.

2. Donor considerations

Upon receiving information regarding a possible donor for a heart transplant, the recipient team considered several essential factors (**Figure 2**) [17], and donor quality assessment is determined first. Once information regarding the donor has been received, donor quality assessment is determined first.

Organic valve disease is considered a contraindication when using a donor organ for heart transplants. It has been reported that certain donor criteria have been expanded safely, but only sporadic cases have been reported in the literature regarding bench repair or replacement of valves before heart transplantation. Of the reports in the last 25 years [6–16], Risher et al. [14] in 1994 were the first to report on mitral commissurotomy of the donor heart before transplantation. However, heart valve disease remains a contraindication for heart donation in most heart transplant centers.

3. Mitral valve abnormalities

Mitral valve bench correction has rarely been performed because of concerns related to the feasibility of repair and durability. The additional ischemic time required to perform valve repair or replacement needs to be taken into account before using a donor heart with valvular dysfunction.

The assessment of mitral valve regurgitation in a donor patient is essential to determine the mechanism, severity, and reversibility of the disease before planning mitral valve repair. A thorough review of the donor echocardiogram should be performed to determine the exact nature and pathology of mitral regurgitation

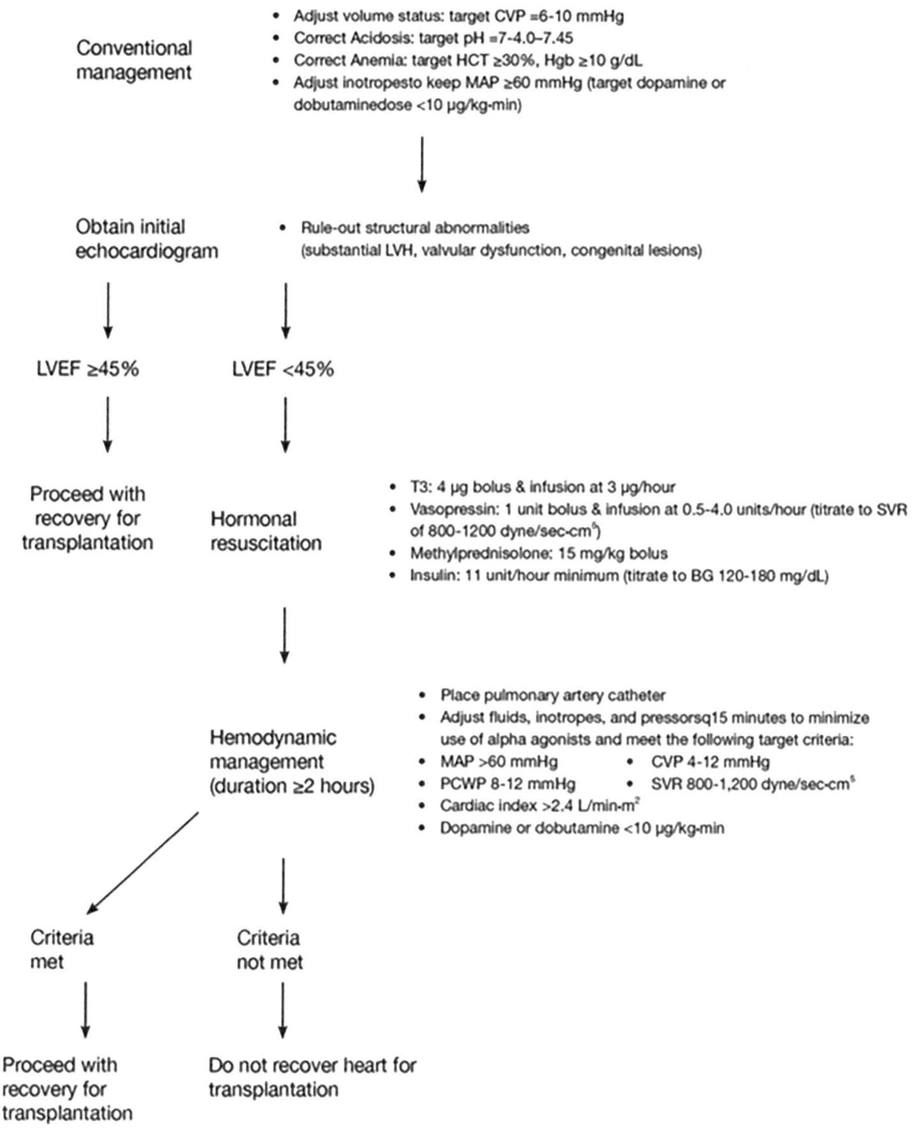

Figure 2.
Guidelines for an algorithm for the management of potential heart donors. CVP: central venous pressure; HCT: hematocrit; Hb: hemoglobin; MAP: mean arterial pressure; LVEF: left ventricular ejection fraction; T3: triiodothyronine; SVR: systemic vascular resistance; BG: blood glucose; and PCWP: pulmonary capillary wedge pressure.

in otherwise acceptable donor hearts. If the mechanism of mitral regurgitation is simple, then bench repair can be performed by increasing the duration of warm ischemia time before transplantation.

However, the evaluation may be compromised by a decrease in afterload resulting from the loss of peripheral vascular tone or inflated by transient ventricular dysfunction [18]. For this purpose, transesophageal echocardiographic evaluation is necessary to understand whether mitral regurgitation is surgically treatable. Therefore, there is sufficient reason to perform bench mitral valve repair without a significant increase in recipient morbidity and mortality. In addition, donor hearts should not show any electrocardiographic or echocardiographic signs of left ventricular hypertrophy (LVH). The authors believe that in some cases, the presence of mitral regurgitation with moderate pulmonary hypertension may be a protective factor as the right ventricle is preconditioned to a high afterload.

4. Aortic valve abnormalities

Only a small number of heart transplants with concomitant aortic valve replacement for moderate-to-severe aortic insufficiency or aortic stenosis have been documented [6, 7, 9, 10, 12, 15]. It has been reported [7] that a bioprosthetic valve is preferred on a predicted average donor heart survival of 10–15 years [2] and the relatively frequent need for endocardial biopsies early after transplantation. The need for warfarin after mechanical valve replacement could lead to frequent bridging and interruption of anticoagulation during scheduled endocardial biopsies. In addition, it was considered that a large bioprosthesis would likely outlast the life of the allograft. When the donor has a bicuspid valve, the donor's aorta carries an increased risk of expansion due to the inherent nature of the bicuspid aortic valve. In younger individuals with normal life expectancy, aortic valve repair may be an excellent alternative since the risk of structural valve deterioration of aortic bioprosthesis is known to be higher in younger patients. Rates of reoperation as high as 50% in 15 years have been reported in 25-year-old patients [19].

If aortic valve replacement is considered for a donor heart, careful evaluation of LVH status and expected ischemic time is mandatory. This is because significant LVH and prolonged ischemic time has been proven to jeopardize transplant outcomes.

The use of donor hearts with LVH has yielded mixed results in terms of recipient outcomes. Kuppahally et al. [20] reported that recipients of donor hearts with LVH ($\geq$ 1.2 cm) had worse survival and a higher incidence of cardiac allograft vasculopathy (CAV). Subsequently, Pinzon et al. [21] reviewed the UNOS database between 2006 and 2010 with almost 3000 recipients and stratified donor hearts into groups without LVH (< 1.1 cm), with mild LVH (1.1–1.3 cm), and with moderate-severe LVH ($\geq$ 1.4 cm). They found similar 30-day and 1-year survival rates across the recipients in all three groups. However, hearts from donors with additional risk factors such as older age or prolonged cold ischemic time ($\geq$4 h) exhibited worse survival [21], suggesting an association between LVH and other donor risk factors. The 2010 ISHLT guidelines for the care of heart transplant recipients state that using donor hearts with LVH (wall thickness < 1.4 cm) and without accompanying electrocardiograms (ECG) findings of LVH may be appropriate (class IIa; level of evidence C) [22]. Thus, the authors suggest that it is reasonable to avoid a donor heart presenting with posterior wall and interventricular septum thickness > 14 mm during diastole. The presence of aortic valve disease (stenosis or insufficiency) in the absence of left ventricular hypertrophy should not preclude donor considerations.

Careful attention must be paid to allograft ischemic time since bench valve surgery requires additional warm ischemic time. Currently, the allograft ischemic time is limited to 4–6 h. In fact, a study utilizing the UNOS database that included over 11,700 patients undergoing heart transplantation reported that ischemic time was an independent risk factor for survival in patients with an ischemic time > 6 hours [OR 1.7 (1.0–2.8), $p < 0.05$] and in patients with an ischemic time between 4 and 6 hours [OR 1.4 (1.3–1.6), $p < 0.05$] [23]. Several reports have shown that longer ischemic time is associated with a higher risk of mortality [24, 25]. Moreover, it has been reported that long cold ischemic time may introduce primary graft dysfunction, CAV, and increased length of stay in intensive care [26, 27]. Conversely, some investigators have demonstrated that a prolonged ischemic time does not negatively impact the 1-year survival following heart transplantation [28, 29]. After the heart allocation policy was revised in the United States [3], it was reported that the mean total allograft ischemic time increased from 3.0 to 3.4 h ($P < 0.001$), with a concurrent increase in median distance between donor and recipient transplant centers from 83 to 216 miles [30]. Therefore, the acceptable maximum allograft ischemic time remains a matter of debate; however, a longer allograft ischemic time is not without risk.

5. Tricuspid valve abnormalities

Heart transplantation is often associated with tricuspid regurgitation (TR). Structural or functional factors can be associated with TR. The biatrial technique of heart transplantation is associated with more TR than the bicaval technique. The incidence of post-transplantation TR has decreased since the introduction of the bicaval anastomosis implantation technique by Yacoub et al. in 1989 [31, 32]. This was believed to be related to the reduced right atrial pressure and preserved right atrial size during the use of a bicaval rather than a biatrial anastomosis technique [33]. Other possible causes of TR include (1) allograft dysfunction with right ventricular dilatation due to poor preservation, reperfusion injury, donor factors, or rejection; (2) pulmonary hypertension; (3) severe donor-recipient size mismatch; and (4) structural damage during endomyocardial biopsy [34–36].

It has been reported that prophylactic tricuspid valve annuloplasty of the donor heart is durable and offers a survival advantage in the perioperative and long-term periods [37, 38]. Considering the simplicity and safety of tricuspid valve annuloplasty and its advantages, there should be a low threshold when considering the procedure as a routine adjunct to heart transplantation.

6. Conclusion

The appropriate utilization of the valve repair/replacement technique with precise assessment of an additional warm ischemic time necessitates careful consideration within each transplant center and each patient potentially willing to accept an allograft with valve disease in the context of the expected allograft cold ischemic time.

Bench valvular replacement or repair of donor allografts during cold ischemia is feasible, and its implementation could enable the use of previously unsalvageable hearts, thus expanding the donor organ pool. Bench valve surgery, combined with proper donor and recipient selection, will enable the expansion of the donor pool to provide high-quality donor allografts that otherwise would have been declined.

Conflict of interest

None.

Author details

Yasuhiro Shudo
Department of Cardiothoracic Surgery, Stanford University School of Medicine, Stanford, CA, United States

*Address all correspondence to: yshudo@stanford.edu

References

[1] Hunt SA, Abraham WT, Chin MH, Feldman AM, Francis GS, Ganiats TG, et al. American College of Cardiology, American Heart Association Task Force on Practice Guidelines, American College of Chest Physicians, International Society for Heart and Lung Transplantation, Heart Rhythm Society. ACC/AHA. 2005 guideline update for the diagnosis and management of chronic heart failure in adults: A report of the American College of Cardiology. Circulation/American Heart Association Task Force on Practice Guidelines. 2005;**112**:e154-e235

[2] Khush KK, Cherikh WS, Chambers DC, et al. The International Thoracic Organ Transplant Registry of the International Society for Heart and Lung Transplantation: Thirty-sixth adult heart transplantation report – 2019; focus theme: Donor and recipient size match. The Journal of Heart and Lung Transplantation. 2019;**38**:1056-1066

[3] US Department of Health and Human Services. Organ Procurement and Transplantation Network. 2021. Available at: https://optn.transplant.hrsa.gov/

[4] Wittwer T, Wahlers T. Marginal donor grafts in heart transplantation: Lessons learned from 25 years of experience. Transplant International. 2008;**21**:113-125

[5] Zaroff JG, Rosengard BR, Armstrong WF, Babcock WD, D'Alessandro A, Dec GW, et al. Consensus Conference Report. Consensus conference report: Maximizing use of organs recovered from the cadaver donor: Cardiac recommendations, March 28-29, 2001, Crystal City. Circulation. 2002;**106**:836-841

[6] Fiore A, Grande AM, Gatti G, et al. Valvular surgery in donor hearts before orthotopic heart transplantation. Archives of Cardiovascular Diseases. 2020;**113**:674-678

[7] Sultan I, Seese L, Lagazzi L, Gleason TG. Concomitant aortic valve replacement with orthotopic heart transplantation. The Journal of Thoracic and Cardiovascular Surgery. 2018;**155**:e151-e152

[8] Prieto D, Antunes P, Antunes MJ. Donor mitral valve repair in cardiac transplantation. Transplantation Proceedings. 2009;**41**:932-934

[9] Saito S, Matsumiya G, Ueno T, et al. Bench replacement of donor aortic valve before orthotopic heart transplantation. The Journal of Heart and Lung Transplantation. 2009;**28**:981-983

[10] Larobina ME, Mariani JA, Rowland MA. Aortic valve replacement for aortic stenosis during orthotopic cardiac transplant. The Annals of Thoracic Surgery. 2008;**86**:1979-1982

[11] Antunes PE, Prieto D, Eugénio L, Antunes MJ. Donor mitral valve repair in cardiac transplantation. The Journal of Thoracic and Cardiovascular Surgery. 2005;**129**:227-228

[12] Navia JL, Atik FA, Marullo A, et al. Bench repair of donor aortic valve with minimal access orthotopic heart transplantation. The Annals of Thoracic Surgery. 2005;**80**:313-315

[13] Massad MG, Smedira NG, Hobbs RE, Hoercher K, Vandervoort P, McCarthy PM. Bench repair of donor mitral valve before heart transplantation. The Annals of Thoracic Surgery. 1996;**61**:1833-1835

[14] Risher WH, Ochsner JL, Van Meter C. Cardiac transplantation after donor mitral valve commissurotomy.

The Annals of Thoracic Surgery. 1994;**57**:221-222

[15] Okamura H, Woo YJ. Ex vivo allograft mitral valve leaflet repair prior to orthotopic heart transplantation. Journal of Cardiac Surgery. 2014;**29**:424-426

[16] Patel M, Vahdat KK, Nathan S, et al. Bioprosthetic aortic valve replacement in a donor heart before orthotopic heart transplantation. Texas Heart Institute Journal. 2017;**44**:135-137

[17] Kilic A, Emani S, Sai-Sudhakar CB, et al. Donor selection in heart transplantation. Journal of Thoracic Disease. 2014;**6**:1097-1104

[18] Zaroff JG, Babcock WD, Shiboski SC, Solinger LL, Rosengard BR. Temporal changes in left ventricular systolic function in heart donors: Results of serial echocardiography. The Journal of Heart and Lung Transplantation. 2003;**22**:383-388

[19] Banbury MK, Cosgrove DM 3rd, White JA, Blackstone EH, Frater RWM, Okies JE. Age and valve size effect on the long-term durability of the Carpentier-Edwards aortic pericardial bioprosthesis. The Annals of Thoracic Surgery. 2001;**72**:753-757

[20] Kuppahally SS, Valantine HA, Weisshaar D, Parekh H, Hung YY, Haddad F, et al. Outcome in cardiac recipients of donor hearts with increased left ventricular wall thickness. American Journal of Transplantation. 2007;**7**:2388-2395

[21] Wever Pinzon OW, Stoddard G, Drakos SG, Gilbert EM, Nativi JN, Budge D, et al. Impact of donor left ventricular hypertrophy on survival after heart transplantation. American Journal of Transplantation. 2011; **11**:2755-2761

[22] Costanzo MR, Dipchand A, Starling R, Anderson A, Chan M, Desai S, et al. The International Society of heart and lung transplantation guidelines for the care of heart transplant recipients. The Journal of Heart and Lung Transplantation. 2010;**29**:914-956

[23] Hong KN, Iribarne A, Worku B, et al. Who is a high-risk recipient? Predicting mortality after heart transplant using pretransplant donor and recipient risk factors. The Annals of Thoracic Surgery. 2011;**92**:520-527

[24] Kilic A, Weiss ES, Allen JG, Conte JV, Shah AS, Baumgartner WA, et al. Simple score to assess the risk of rejection after orthotopic heart transplantation. Circulation. 2012;**125**:3013-3021

[25] Mitropoulos FA, Odim J, Marelli D, et al. Outcome of hearts with cold ischemic time greater than 300 minutes. A case-matched study. European Journal of Cardio-Thoracic Surgery. 2005;**28**:143-148

[26] Russo MJ, Chen JM, Sorabella RA, et al. The effect of ischemic time on survival after heart transplantation varies by donor age: An analysis of the United Network for Organ Sharing database. The Journal of Thoracic and Cardiovascular Surgery. 2007;**133**:554-559

[27] Derek M, Yellon D, Hausenloy DJ. Myocardial perfusion injury. The New England Journal of Medicine. 2007;**357**:1121-1135

[28] Morgan JA, John R, Weinberg AD, et al. Prolonged donor ischemic time does not adversely affect the long-term survival in adult patients undergoing cardiac transplantation. The Journal of Thoracic and Cardiovascular Surgery. 2003;**126**:1624-1633

[29] Currie ME, Shudo Y, Woo YJ. Successful outcome following orthotopic heart transplantation with a donor half way across the country.

Transplantation Proceedings. 2018;**50**:4062-4063

[30] Goff RR, Uccellini K, Lindblad K, Hall S, Davies R, Farr M, et al. A change of heart: Preliminary results of the US 2018 adult heart allocation revision. American Journal of Transplantation. 2020;**20**:2781-2790

[31] Yacoub M, Mankad P, Ledingham S. Donor procurement and surgical techniques for cardiac transplantation. Seminars in Thoracic and Cardiovascular Surgery. 1990;**2**:153-161

[32] Aziz T, Burgess M, Khafagy R, Wynn Hann A, Campbell C, Rahman A, et al. Bicaval and standard techniques in orthotopic heart transplantation: Medium-term experience in cardiac performance and survival. The Journal of Thoracic and Cardiovascular Surgery. 1999;**118**:115-122

[33] Jacob S, Sellke F. Is bicaval orthotopic heart transplantation superior to the biatrial technique? Interactive Cardiovascular and Thoracic Surgery. 2009;**9**:333-342

[34] Kwon MH, Shemin RJ. Tricuspid valve regurgitation after heart transplantation. Annals of Cardiothoracic Surgery. 2017;**6**:270-274

[35] Chan MC, Giannetti N, Kato T, Kornbluth M, Oyer P, Valantine HA, et al. Severe tricuspid regurgitation after heart transplantation. The Journal of Heart and Lung Transplantation. 2001;**20**:709-717

[36] Nguyen V, Cantarovich M, Cecere R, Giannetti N. Tricuspid regurgitation after cardiac transplantation: How many biopsies are too many? The Journal of Heart and Lung Transplantation. 2005;**24**(7):S227-S231

[37] Jeevanandam V, Russell H, Mather P, Furukawa S, Anderson A, Raman J. Donor tricuspid annuloplasty during orthotopic heart transplantation: Long-term results of a prospective controlled study. The Annals of Thoracic Surgery. Dec 2006;**82**:2089-2095

[38] Fiorelli AI, Oliveira JL, Santos RH, Coelho GB, Oliveira AS, Lourenço-Filho DD, et al. Can tricuspid annuloplasty of the donor heart reduce valve insufficiency following cardiac transplantation with bicaval anastomosis? Heart Surgery Forum. 2010;**13**:E168-E171